ACSM's
Health-Related Physical Fitness
Assessment Manual
FOURTH EDITION

EDITOR

Leonard A. Kaminsky, PhD, FACSM
Coordinator, Clinical Exercise Physiology Program
Human Performance Laboratory
Ball State University
Muncie, Indiana

ACSM's
Health-Related Physical Fitness
Assessment Manual

FOURTH EDITION

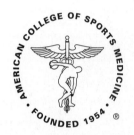

AMERICAN COLLEGE
OF SPORTS MEDICINE

Wolters Kluwer | Lippincott Williams & Wilkins
Health

Publisher: Chris Johnson
Acquisitions Editor: Emily Lupash
Product Director: Eric Branger
Senior Product Manager: Heather A. Rybacki
Product Manager: Michael Marino
Production Project Manager: Marian Bellus
Marketing Manager: Sarah Schuessler
Manufacturing Coordinator: Margie Orzech-Zeranko
Design Coordinator: Doug Smock
ACSM Publications Committee Chair: Walter R. Thompson, PhD, FACSM, FAACVPR
ACSM Group Publisher: Kerry O'Rourke
Compositor: Absolute Service, Inc.

Fourth Edition

351 West Camden Street   Two Commerce Square
Baltimore, MD 21201   2001 Market Street
                                Philadelphia, PA 19103

Printed in China

9 8 7 6 5 4 3 2 1

Library of Congress Cataloging-in-Publication Data

ACSM's health-related physical fitness assessment manual. — 4th ed. / editor, Leonard A. Kaminsky ; American College of Sports Medicine.
   p. ; cm.
  Health-related physical fitness assessment manual
  Companion to: ACSM's guidelines for exercise testing and prescription. 9th ed. 2013.
  Includes bibliographical references and index.
  ISBN 978-1-4511-1568-0
  I. Kaminsky, Leonard A., 1955- II. American College of Sports Medicine. III. American College of Sports Medicine. ACSM's guidelines for exercise testing and prescription. IV. Title: Health-related physical fitness assessment manual.
  [DNLM: 1. Physical Fitness—Guideline. 2. Exercise Test—standards—Guideline. 3. Physical Endurance—Guideline. 4. Physical Examination—standards—Guideline. QT 255]

  615.8'2—dc23

                                                                    2012043393

DISCLAIMER

    Care has been taken to confirm the accuracy of the information present and to describe generally accepted practices. However, the authors, editors, and publisher are not responsible for errors or omissions or for any consequences from application of the information in this book and make no warranty, expressed or implied, with respect to the currency, completeness, or accuracy of the contents of the publication. Application of this information in a particular situation remains the professional responsibility of the practitioner; the clinical treatments described and recommended may not be considered absolute and universal recommendations.
    The authors, editors, and publisher have exerted every effort to ensure that drug selection and dosage set forth in this text are in accordance with the current recommendations and practice at the time of publication. However, in view of ongoing research, changes in government regulations, and the constant flow of information relating to drug therapy and drug reactions, the reader is urged to check the package insert for each drug for any change in indications and dosage and for added warnings and precautions. This is particularly important when the recommended agent is a new or infrequently employed drug.
    Some drugs and medical devices presented in this publication have Food and Drug Administration (FDA) clearance for limited use in restricted research settings. It is the responsibility of the health care provider to ascertain the FDA status of each drug or device planned for use in their clinical practice.

To purchase additional copies of this book, call our customer service department at (800) 638-3030 or fax orders to (301) 223-2320. International customers should call (301) 223-2300.

Visit Lippincott Williams & Wilkins on the Internet: http://www.lww.com. Lippincott Williams & Wilkins customer service representatives are available from 8:30 am to 6:00 pm, EST.

For more information concerning American College of Sports Medicine certification and suggested preparatory materials, call (800) 486-5643 or visit the American College of Sports Medicine Website at www.acsm.org.

Preface

The American College of Sports Medicine has long been a leader in advocating the health benefits associated with a physically active lifestyle. When, in October 2008, the U.S. Department of Health and Human Services released the first ever Federal policy report, *Physical Activity Guidelines for Americans*, recognition of the importance of performing regular physical activity for good health took a major leap forward (www.health.gov/PAguidelines/). Clinicians, public health professionals, and allied health professionals will now, more than ever, need the expertise of those trained and knowledgeable of how to prescribe physical activity/exercise and how to subsequently measure the effects of these programs. As stated in *Chapter 1* of this Manual, *physical fitness is the measureable outcome of a person's physical activity and exercise habits.* Thus, it is essential that exercise professionals remain well versed in the methods of health-related physical fitness assessment and the interpretation of the results of these assessments. The importance of physical fitness assessment is supported by three recent reports. Readers of this manual are encouraged to review the literature summary by Arena, Myers, and Guazzi[1] that makes a compelling case for including aerobic exercise testing results as a key vital sign in clinical practice. Likewise, reports on the importance of body composition assessment both to measure fat[2] and muscle[3] mass should be read.

This fourth edition of the *ACSM's Health-Related Physical Fitness Assessment Manual* provides important updates consistent with the most current resource information available on measuring physical fitness. For this edition, all photographs were improved to provide significantly more detail and clearer presentation of important physical fitness measurement–related concepts. The intent of this Manual remains to provide a comprehensive overview of why and how to perform assessments of the five health-related components of physical fitness — namely, body composition, muscular strength, muscular endurance, flexibility, and cardiorespiratory fitness. This Manual is an extension of assessment principles covered in the *ACSM Guidelines for Exercise Testing and Prescription, Ninth Edition* and includes many of the summary tables and figures from the *Guidelines*. After mastering the assessment procedures, the users of this Manual are encouraged to interpret the results with a clear understanding of the specific methodological limitations that exist for some of the procedures.

The value of physical fitness assessment results as a key health indicator is now well accepted. This Manual provides the foundational key concepts and methods of health-related physical fitness assessment for all exercise science and allied health professionals.

---

[1]Arena R, Myers J, Guazzi M. The future of aerobic exercise testing in clinical practice: is it the ultimate vital sign? *Future Cardiol.* 2010;6:325–42.

[2]Cornier MA, Després JP, Davis N, et al. Assessing adiposity: a scientific statement from the American Heart Association. *Circulation.* 2011;124:1996–2019.

[3]Cruz-Jentoft AJ, Baeyens JP, Bauer JM, et al. Sarcopenia: European consensus on definition and diagnosis: Report of the European Working Group on sarcopenia in older people. *Age Ageing.* 2010;39:412–23.

FEATURES

....

- Reorganized and expanded information, including discussion of unique assessment principles and the major limitations of some assessment methods
- Step-by-step instructions for assessment of health-related physical fitness and resources for interpretation of test results
- Updated references to *ACSM's Guidelines for Exercise Testing and Prescription, Ninth Edition*
- More than 110 boxes, tables, and figures to help the reader understand the concepts of health-related physical fitness
- Case study analysis at the conclusion of each assessment chapter and suggested laboratory activities to help students master the concepts of health-related physical fitness

SUPPLEMENTAL MATERIALS

....

Supplemental materials for students and instructors are available at http://thepoint.lww.com/activate.

Instructors can access the following:

- PowerPoint Lecture Outlines
- Image Bank, including all figures and tables from the text
- Full Text Online
- Data Collection Forms

Students can also access the Full Text Online and Data Collection Forms.

Acknowledgments

When writing acknowledgments, one always runs the risk of omitting the mention of someone who has contributed. I am truly appreciative to all who provided support and assistance to the development of the fourth edition of this Manual. With that being said, I do want to specifically acknowledge and thank the following individuals and groups.

Thanks to Dr. Greg Dwyer, who, through his teaching of fitness assessment to undergraduate Exercise Science students, recognized the need for a comprehensive manual of health-related physical fitness assessment. Greg, along with his coeditor Dr. Shala Davis, produced the first two editions of this Manual. All of us who teach and the students who learn health-related physical fitness assessment are indebted to Dr. Dwyer and Dr. Davis.

I appreciate all of the members of the American College of Sports Medicine who volunteer their time to our professional organization. I especially extend my gratitude to Dr. Walt Thompson, Chair of the Publications Committee, and the ACSM member reviewers for sharing their expertise to help improve this fourth edition. I wish to thank the editorial group of the ninth edition of *ACSM's Guidelines for Exercise Testing and Prescription* for their cooperation in sharing materials that are incorporated in this Manual. My gratitude is also extended to the professional staff of the American College of Sports Medicine, particularly Kerrie O'Rourke, for her support in the development of publications for this organization.

Thanks to the talented and hardworking staff at Wolters Kluwer Health/Lippincott Williams & Wilkins whom I have worked with now on four separate ACSM publications. I particularly want to extend my gratitude to Michael Marino and Emily Lupash for their assistance throughout this project.

Thanks to my professional colleagues at Ball State University's Human Performance Laboratory, especially Lynn Clark, for all of their support. I also extend my appreciation to all the excellent graduate students whom I have had the honor of working with as they complete their training in Clinical Exercise Physiology at Ball State University. Every day, you are doing the important work with the public to help them understand the importance of physical fitness and applying it to improve their health.

I dedicate this work to those whom were most influential in my professional training: Dr. Peter Gifford, Dr. Ronald Knowlton, Dr. Noel Nequin, Dr. Dave Costill, Dr. Bud Getchell, Dr. Mitch Whaley, and Dr. Pete Brubaker. You have all done so much for our profession and have truly been an inspiration to me and many others.

And finally, thank you to my wife Mary and my daughters Lauren and Bonnie for your continuing love and support. I also thank them for their behind-the-scenes assistance in support of the production of this manual.

Reviewers

Mary Jo Adams
Illinois State University
Normal, Illinois

Robert E. Alman, II, EdD
Indiana University of Pennsylvania
Indiana, Pennsylvania

Stephen D. Ball, PhD
University of Missouri
Columbia, Missouri

Stacey Beam
Coastal Carolina University
Conway, South Carolina

Steve Burns
University of Central Missouri
Warrensburg, Missouri

Karen K. Dennis
Illinois State University
Normal, Illinois

Teresa C. Fitts, DPE
Westfield State University
Westfield, Massachusetts

Warren Franke
Iowa State University
Ames, Iowa

Peter Grandjean, PhD, FACSM
Baylor University
Waco, Texas

Kim Henige
California State University, Northridge
Los Angeles, California

Greg K. Kandt, EdD
Fort Hays State University
Hays, Kansas

Raymond M. Kraus, PhD
Elmhurst College
Elmhurst, Illinois

Jeff Lynn
Slippery Rock University
Slippery Rock, Pennsylvania

Peter M. Magyari, PhD
University of North Florida
Jacksonville, Florida

Reid A. Perry
Globe University
Woodbury, Minnesota

James Schoffstall
Liberty University
Lynchburg, Virginia

Julie A. Snyder
Keiser University
Port St. Lucie, Florida

Lucille Sternburgh, MS
Beaumont Health & Wellness Center
Rochester Hills, Michigan

Contents

1

Introduction

DEFINING HEALTH-RELATED PHYSICAL FITNESS

The purpose of *ACSM's Health-Related Physical Fitness Assessment Manual* is to provide a thorough overview of assessments of health-related physical fitness (HRPF). Physical fitness has been described in many different ways, as noted in *Table 1.1*, and thus, confusion regarding the specific meaning of this common term can easily occur. Indeed, the terms physical fitness, health-related physical fitness, exercise, and physical activity, although distinct and unique, are oftentimes used incorrectly due to their interrelated nature.

Because it is important for allied health professionals to have a clear understanding of the exact meaning of the term **physical fitness**, the U.S. Centers for Disease Control and Prevention (CDC) established the following standard definition in 1985: ". . . a set of attributes or characteristics that people have or achieve that relates to the ability to perform physical activity" (2).

Health-related physical fitness, an additional and more specific term, has been defined by the President's Council on Physical Fitness as consisting of "those specific components of physical fitness that have a relationship with good health" (7). Additionally, there are other components of physical fitness such as agility, balance, coordination, power, speed, and reaction time that are important for what is called sport- or skill-related physical fitness.

People achieve physical fitness through **exercise**, which the CDC defines as ". . . a subcategory of physical activity that is planned, structured, repetitive and purposive in the sense that improvement or maintenance of one or more components of physical fitness is the objective" (10).

TABLE 1.1. Definitions of Physical Fitness

Source	Definition
Getchell (3)	Physical fitness is the capability of the heart, blood vessels, lungs, and muscles to perform at optimal efficiency.
Miller et al. (5)	General physical fitness is a state of ability to perform sustained physical work characterized by an effective integration of cardiorespiratory endurance, strength, flexibility, coordination, and body composition.
President's Council on Physical Fitness and Sports Research Digests (7)	Physical fitness is the ability to carry out daily tasks with vigor and alertness without undue fatigue and with ample energy to enjoy leisure-time pursuits and respond to emergencies.

The *ACSM's Guidelines for Exercise Testing and Prescription, Ninth Edition (GETP9)* provides specific guidelines for exercise training to improve HRPF.

Physical activity has been shown to be related to health and therefore is a term that must be clearly defined and understood. The CDC defines **physical activity** as "any bodily movement produced by the contraction of skeletal muscles that increases energy expenditure above a basal level" (10).

It is important to use all the cited terms correctly and have a clear understanding that physical fitness is a measurable set of characteristics determined by the exercise habits of an individual. Certainly, genetics also plays a role in the level of physical fitness one can achieve. Those with the highest levels of physical fitness have the optimal genetic makeup and have maximized their exercise training.

COMPONENTS OF HEALTH-RELATED PHYSICAL FITNESS

The American College of Sports Medicine (ACSM) has been a leader in setting guidelines for the assessment of physical fitness, particularly HRPF. Five measurable components of HRPF are depicted in *Figure 1.1*.

Cardiorespiratory endurance refers to the ability of the circulatory and the respiratory systems to supply oxygen during sustained physical activity. **Cardiorespiratory fitness** is related to the ability to perform large-muscle, dynamic, moderate-to-high intensity exercise for prolonged periods. The methods of assessment of cardiorespiratory fitness are provided in *Chapters 7* and *8* of this manual.

Body composition refers to the relative amount or percentage of different types of body tissue (bone, fat, muscle) that are related to health. The most common health-related measure is that of total body fat percentage; however, it should be noted that there are no established criterion values for this measure related to health

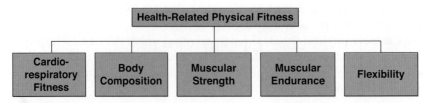

■ **FIGURE 1.1.** Health-related physical fitness is not a single entity, but rather a sum of five measurable components.

parameters. The methods used to assess body composition are provided in *Chapter 4* of this manual.

Muscular strength is related to the ability to perform activities that require high levels of muscular force. *Chapter 5* of this manual has specific measurement information on muscular strength.

Muscular endurance is the ability of a muscle group to execute repeated contractions over a period of time sufficient to cause muscular fatigue or to maintain a specific percentage of the maximum voluntary contraction for a prolonged period of time. *Chapter 5* of this manual has specific measurement information on muscular endurance.

Note: To better describe their integrated status, muscular strength and muscular endurance can be combined into one component of HRPF termed **muscular fitness**.

Flexibility is the ability to move a joint through its complete range of movement. *Chapter 6* of this manual has specific measurement information on flexibility. *Figure 1.2* displays one type of assessment of flexibility.

Even though an individual's appearance or exercise habits may be viewed as evidence of physical fitness and health, in reality, there is not one overall measure of physical fitness. Often, regular exercisers spend most of their time training only one component of physical fitness. For example, the person who runs long distances 6 d $\cdot$ wk^{-1} may be considered "physically fit" (and indeed may be in terms of cardiorespiratory fitness); however, this person is often below average in terms of muscular strength and flexibility. Likewise, it is common for someone who performs high levels of resistance training as the sole form of exercise to be viewed as physically fit (and indeed may be in terms of muscular strength and muscular endurance); however, this person is often below average in terms of cardiorespiratory fitness and flexibility. Thus, it is important to view HRPF as an integration of the five components.

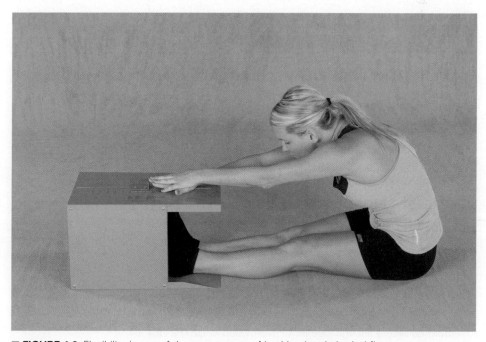

■ **FIGURE 1.2.** Flexibility is one of the components of health-related physical fitness.

THE IMPORTANCE OF MEASURING HEALTH-RELATED PHYSICAL FITNESS

THE RELATIONSHIP OF PHYSICAL FITNESS TO HEALTH

Throughout history, humans have broadly recognized the relationship between physical fitness and health. In ancient China, records of organized exercise as a means of health promotion date from 2500 B.C., and there is much evidence that the ancient Greeks "emphasized the importance of physical well-being, fitness and a healthy lifestyle" (4). Yet, systematic investigation and research of this relationship didn't begin until the 1960s. From that time forward, scientific literature has firmly established the relationship between physical activity and health. In 1996, this new body of research served as a basis for a notable comprehensive report from the U.S. Surgeon General entitled *Physical Activity and Health* (12).

This report by the U.S. Surgeon General provided an extensive review of research demonstrating various health-related benefits obtained from physical activity. The report also emphasized what is termed the *dose-response* relationship. The *dose* in this term refers to the amount of physical activity and/or exercise, whereas the *response* references the resultant health outcome. Although the evidence is quite clear that exercise doses result in many health benefits (as noted in *Box 1.1*), the exact minimal dose of physical activity and/or exercise required to produce health benefits is not yet clearly discerned. The *2008 Physical Activity Guidelines for Americans*, produced by the U.S. Department of Health and Human Services, represents another recent comprehensive report based on major research findings regarding the relationship between physical activity and health (11). This publication is an essential resource for all exercise professionals. This report provides the following summary suggestions regarding duration and intensity of physical activity:

- All adults should avoid inactivity. Some physical activity is better than none.
- Both aerobic (endurance) and muscle-strengthening (resistance) physical activity are beneficial.

BOX 1.1   Some Benefits of Regular Physical Activity and/or Exercise

IMPROVEMENT IN CARDIOVASCULAR AND RESPIRATORY FUNCTION
- Increased maximal oxygen uptake resulting from both central and peripheral adaptations
- Decreased heart rate and blood pressure at a given submaximal intensity

REDUCTION IN CARDIOVASCULAR DISEASE RISK FACTORS
- Reduced resting systolic/diastolic pressures
- Increased serum high-density lipoprotein cholesterol and decreased serum triglycerides

DECREASED MORBIDITY AND MORTALITY
- Higher activity and/or fitness levels are associated with lower incidence rates for combined cardiovascular diseases, coronary artery disease, stroke, and many other chronic diseases

OTHER BENEFITS
- Decreased anxiety and depression
- Improved cognitive function

A more complete listing of benefits is provided in *GETP9 Box 1.4*.

- For substantial health benefits, adults should do at least 150 min (2 h and 30 min) a week of moderate intensity, or 75 min (1 h and 15 min) a week of vigorous intensity aerobic physical activity, or an equivalent combination of moderate and vigorous intensity, aerobic activity.
- For additional and more extensive health benefits, adults should increase their aerobic physical activity to 300 min (5 h) a week of moderate intensity, or 150 min a week (2 h and 30 min) of vigorous intensity, aerobic physical activity, or an equivalent combination of moderate and vigorous intensity, aerobic physical activity.
- Adults should also do muscle-strengthening activities that are moderate or high intensity and involve all major muscle groups on 2 or more days a week because these activities provide additional health benefits.

Additionally, in 2011, the ACSM published a revised position stand "to provide scientific evidence-based recommendations to health and fitness professionals in the development of individualized exercise prescriptions for apparently healthy adults of all ages" (1). Remember that it is exercise that promotes the maintenance or improvement in physical fitness. In other words, physical fitness is the measurable outcome of a person's physical activity and exercise habits. Thus, many health care providers are increasingly valuing the measurement of HRPF.

Among the important reasons for assessing HRPF, as cited in the *ACSM's GETP9*, are the following:

- *Educating participants about their present health-related fitness status relative to health-related standards and age- and sex-matched norms.* Good health care for an individual includes knowing important personal health-related information such as one's cholesterol level and blood pressure. Similarly, knowledge of HRPF measurements would support optimizing personal health.
- *Providing data that are helpful in the development of individualized exercise prescriptions to address all health/fitness components.* Maintenance or improvement in the different components of HRPF requires different types of exercise training. Thus, although there are some generalized exercise recommendations for good health, the exercise prescription can and should be tailored to the specific needs and goals of the individual. This is best achieved by having current HRPF measurements.
- *Collecting baseline and follow-up data that allow evaluation of progress by exercise program participants.* Other personal health information, such as cholesterol and blood pressure, is tracked over time. Similarly, measuring HRPF periodically can aid an individual in managing personal health. Measurements through time can also help identify whether training program modifications need to be made to improve some components of HRPF while maintaining desired levels of the other components of HRPF.
- *Motivating participants by establishing reasonable and attainable fitness goals.* Knowing one's HRPF measures provides a basis for individualizing a physical fitness program. Periodic assessments allow for tracking progress toward attainment of established goals.

THE RELATIONSHIP OF PHYSICAL FITNESS TO FUNCTION

It has been well recognized that many aspects of sport performance are related to physical fitness. Indeed, there are several sport-related physical fitness components such as power, agility, and balance that can be assessed. Although not necessarily related to a specific performance outcome, the components of HRPF are now being recognized as important to the function of everyday tasks and leisure-time pursuits. For example, consider a household

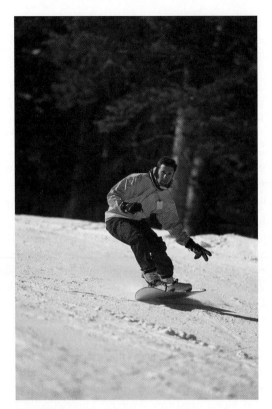

■ **FIGURE 1.3.** People who are physically fit are capable of performing both occupational and recreational activities throughout their lifetimes.

task such as a landscaping project at home that will require lifting bags that could weigh between 10 and 50 lb, repeatedly shoveling materials into a wheelbarrow, and bending and reaching. These tasks require sufficient levels of muscular strength, muscular endurance, and flexibility. Also, consider the opportunity to travel with a group that will be taking a camping trip to a scenic wilderness location. This experience will involve a fair degree of hiking, and the ability to perform this activity will require a certain level of cardiorespiratory fitness and muscular endurance and will be influenced by body composition.

These are only two examples of how HRPF is related to function. Certainly, the performance of many of the activities of daily living depends on one's physical fitness level, and this becomes even more apparent as one ages. *Figure 1.3* shows an example of a recreational activity that can be performed throughout one's lifetime if one maintains an adequate level of HRPF.

FUNDAMENTAL PRINCIPLES OF ASSESSMENT

For each of the components of HRPF, there are various assessment methods that can be used. *Chapters 4–8* of this manual will provide an overview of assessment procedures and interpretations for each of the components of HRPF. However, regardless of which component of HRPF is assessed, there are fundamental principles that should be applied in performing physical fitness assessments.

A SPECIFIC ASSESSMENT OBJECTIVE

A clear purpose should be identified prior to performing the assessment. A list of important reasons for performing HRPF measurements is provided on the previous page. Both the client and the physical fitness professional should have a clear understanding of the objective of the assessment. Knowing this objective will ensure the selection of the most appropriate procedure.

THE GOLD STANDARD (TRUE MEASURE)

A general principle in assessment is that one test is considered the criterion test or gold standard; that is, it is considered the definitive or true measure. This does not necessarily mean that it is a perfect test, but that it is considered the best test that exists for measuring a specific variable. Although ideal, the gold standard test may not always be used owing to several different circumstances such as the need for expensive equipment and trained personnel, the requirement of extensive time, and the increased risk level to the client.

Error of Measurement

If the use of the gold standard test is not feasible, other tests can be employed to estimate the variable of interest. This typically leads to some level of inaccuracy. For most physiologic variables, such as measures of HRPF, the distribution of errors in measurement follows that of the normal bell curve, as depicted in *Figure 1.4*. When expressing a measurement value from an estimation-type test, the value should include the error range. This is typically expressed as ± 1 standard deviation from the mean, or in prediction equations, the standard error of estimate (SEE). For example, if a test reported a mean value of 50 with a standard deviation of 5 (50 $\pm$ 5), this means that if there were 100 cases with a value estimated to be 50, 68 of those cases would have an actual value between 45 and 55, 95 of the cases would have an actual value between 40 and 60, and five cases would have values either <40 or >60. Specifics about measurement errors for different HRPF tests will be provided in *Chapters 4–8*. Thus, it is essential for the physical fitness professional to understand the amount of error in measurement when using indirect tests to estimate an HRPF component.

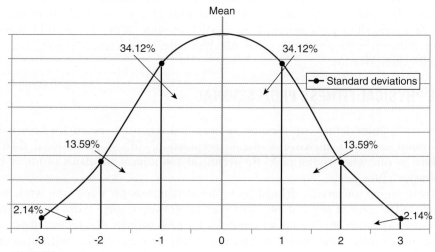

■ **FIGURE 1.4.** The characteristics of the normal bell curve.

EQUIPMENT CALIBRATION

Some instruments or equipment employed in assessments provide accurate measurements every time if used correctly. For example, a wall-mounted stadiometer is a stable device that measures distance accurately. However, a device such as a weight scale may over time produce different readings for standard weight. To ensure the accuracy of the reading, the device must be calibrated prior to the testing session and properly adjusted to produce an accurate reading.

STANDARDIZATION

Another fundamental principle for assessment involves following standardized procedures. Many factors can cause variability in a measurement, so applying uniform standards reduces or eliminates the sources of variability. These may include pretest instructions that may extend to the time 24 h prior to the test (*e.g.*, no vigorous exercise on the day prior to the test) and the environmental conditions of the fitness testing facility (*e.g.*, temperature between 20° C and 24° C).

INTERPRETATION ISSUES

Ideally, there exists one standard that can be used to interpret the results of a test. For example, it is well accepted that in a health assessment that includes a total cholesterol measurement, the results are interpreted with the values established by the National Cholesterol Education Program (NCEP) (6). Unfortunately, no national set of standards has been established for HRPF assessment interpretation.

Types of Standards

There are two basic types of standards: criterion-referenced and normative. **Criterion-referenced standards** are a set of scores that classify the result as desirable (or above or below desirable) based on some external criteria, such as the betterment of health. A group of experts has determined what is desirable. Criterion-referenced standards often use adjectives such as "excellent" or "poor" in classifying test results. **Normative standards**, sometimes referred to as norms, are based on the past performance of groups of individuals with similar characteristics (*e.g.*, age, gender). Thus, with normative standards, a comparison is made between the client's performance and the performance of similar individuals. The data interpretation classifications often use a percentile score such as 90th, 50th, etc. In HRPF assessment, there are more normative standards than criterion-referenced standards available for interpretation.

THE PHYSICAL FITNESS PROFESSIONAL

Merriam-Webster defines a profession as "a calling requiring specialized knowledge and often long and intensive academic preparation" (8). A professional then is defined as one who "conforms to the technical and ethical standards of his or her profession" (9).

There are no universally defined professional standards for those who work with people in the areas of physical fitness or exercise. However, some states have pursued licensure legislation that would set standards for professionals that provide these services. Additionally, some employers have voluntarily set standards for individuals they hire to perform physical fitness assessments or to supervise exercise programs.

ACADEMIC TRAINING

For many years, universities have offered degrees focused on exercise, many of these originating from physical education programs. The exact title of the degree (*e.g.*, Exercise Physiology, Exercise Science, Kinesiology) is unique to the institution, as is the required curriculum. Degrees are offered at the associate, bachelor's, master's, and doctoral levels. Some professional organizations, including ACSM, have initiated efforts to support accreditation of academic programs that offer degree programs in Exercise Science.

CREDENTIALS

Many people who work in the area of physical fitness assessment and/or in providing exercise program services obtain a certification, usually from a professional organization, which attests that they have achieved a minimal level of knowledge and/or competency. Although there are literally hundreds of different organizations and groups that offer some form of certification related to physical fitness assessment and/or exercise services, ACSM has been a leader in providing these types of certifications. The Institute for Credentialing Excellence created the National Commission for Certifying Agencies (NCCA) to demonstrate that certification programs have met minimal standards for professional competence. Presently, ACSM offers five different types of NCAA accredited certifications, with prerequisite requirements ranging from being 18 yr old with a high school degree and current cardiopulmonary resuscitation (CPR) and automated external defibrillator (AED) certification (ACSM Certified Group Exercise Instructor^SM) to having a graduate degree in Clinical Exercise Physiology with a minimum of 600 h of clinical work experience (ACSM Registered Clinical Exercise Physiologist®). *Appendix D* of the *ACSM's GETP9* provides detailed information about these ACSM certifications.

REFERENCES

1. American College of Sports Medicine. Position stand: quantity and quality of exercise for developing and maintaining cardiorespiratory, musculoskeletal, and neuromuscular fitness in apparently healthy adults: guidance for prescribing exercise. *Med Sci Sports Exerc*. 2011;43(7):1334–59.
2. Caspersen CJ, Powell KE, Christenson GM. Physical activity, exercise, and physical fitness: definitions and distinctions for health-related research. *Public Health Rep*. 1985;100(2):126–31.
3. Getchell B. *Physical Fitness: A Way of Life*. 4th ed. New York (NY): Macmillan Publishing Co.; 1992. 348 p.
4. MacAuley D. A history of physical activity, health and medicine. *J R Soc Med*. 1994;87:32.
5. Miller AJ, Grais IM, Winslow E, Kaminsky LA. The definition of physical fitness. *J Sports Med Phys Fitness*. 1991;31:639–40.
6. National Cholesterol Education Program. *Third Report of the National Cholesterol Education Program (NCEP) Expert Panel on Detection, Evaluation, and Treatment of High Blood Cholesterol in Adults (Adult Treatment Panel III)*. NIH Publication No. 02-5215. Washington, DC: National Institutes of Health; 2002. 284 p.
7. President's Council on Physical Fitness and Sports Research Digests. Definitions: Health, fitness and physical activity [Internet]. Updated 2008 April 23. [cited 2011 Jul 6]. Available from: www.fitness.gov/publications/digests/digest_mar2000.html
8. "Profession," Merriam-Webster.com [Internet]. 2011 [cited 2011 Jul 6]. Available from: www.merriam-webster.com/dictionary/profession
9. "Professional," Merriam-Webster.com [Internet]. 2011 [cited 2011 Jul 6]. Available from: www.merriam-webster.com/dictionary/professional
10. U.S. Centers for Disease Control and Prevention. *Physical Activity for Everyone: Glossary of Terms* [Internet]. 2011 [cited 2011 Jul 6]. Available from: www.cdc.gov/physicalactivity/everyone/glossary
11. U.S. Department of Health and Human Services. *2008 Physical Activity Guidelines for Americans*. ODPHP publication U0036 [Internet]. 2008 [cited 2011 Jul 6]. Available from: www.health.gov/paguidelines
12. U.S. Department of Health and Human Services. *Physical Activity and Health: A Report of the Surgeon General*. Atlanta, GA: U.S. Department of Health and Human Services, Centers for Disease Control and Prevention, National Center for Chronic Disease Prevention and Health Promotion; 1996. 278 p.

RATIONALE FOR PREASSESSMENT SCREENING

Health-related physical fitness (HRPF) assessment procedures range from assessments, which require no exercise, to those necessitating vigorous or even maximal physical exertion. The associated risks of conducting the assessments range from no risk to serious risk. If the assessments were limited to the nonexercise procedures (*e.g.*, a skinfold measurement for body composition), there would be no need to perform a preassessment screening. However, because there are risks of both cardiovascular and musculoskeletal injuries associated with exercise, then an HRPF assessment requiring exercise will also require a preassessment screening. The risks are related to both the intensity of the exercise and the activity habits of the client. *ACSM's Guidelines for Exercise Testing and Prescription, Ninth Edition (GETP9)* emphasizes this point stating, "The risk of an exercise related event such as sudden cardiac death or acute MI is greatest in those individuals performing unaccustomed physical activity, and is greatest with vigorous intensity, physical activity." More specific information about cardiovascular risks associated with exercise resides in *Chapter 1* of the *ACSM's GETP9*, with summarized data about event rates found in that text's *Tables 1.4, 1.5,* and *1.6.* Similarly, the risks of musculoskeletal injuries are greater in those individuals with known musculoskeletal diseases or previous injuries as well as those who are inactive. It is therefore critical to know the health and activity history of all individuals who will be performing HRPF assessments involving exercise.

INFORMED CONSENT

The first step in the process of HRPF assessment is completion of the informed consent. Therefore, the first contact most individuals have with a program is with the person who administers the informed consent and conducts the risk classification screening. A client's impression of a program may thus depend on this first contact with the staff. Thinking about fitness testing may create anxiety in the client, and the test results may create other unpleasant feelings. Every effort should be made to help the client relax and focus on the beneficial information afforded from the results of the HRPF assessment. Although the exact approach may vary somewhat depending on the client's personality, performing this initial stage of the assessment with calm professionalism is recommended.

Completion of the informed consent must precede the health risk appraisal because determination of the health risk status will require the exchange of private health information and may require procedures that involve physical risk (*e.g.*, blood testing). Additionally, if the HRPF assessment requires exercise, there are risks involved.

The essential steps in executing the informed consent are the following:

- Explaining the purpose of the assessments
- Describing the procedures to be used
- Describing the risks and discomforts associated with the assessments
- Describing the benefits obtained from the assessments
- Describing alternatives (if any)
- Describing the responsibilities required of the client
- Encouraging the client to ask questions at any time
- Explaining how data will be handled (confidentiality)
- Explaining that the client can withdraw his or her consent and stop the assessment process at any time

An example of an informed consent form is provided in *Box 2.1*; however, there are many variations of informed consent forms available from different sources. All professionals performing assessments should take the time to find a standard form that closely matches a given facility's needs and assessments. Modifications to the form can be made to fit specific needs of the HRPF assessment program, and it is recommended that legal counsel review the final form to limit the chances of legal liability. Finally, it is essential that different informed consent forms be used for each different component of a program (*i.e.*, assessments and exercise programs).

THE INFORMED CONSENT PROCESS

The informed consent is not just a form requiring a signature. Rather, it is a process of documentation that attests to the fact that clear communications have taken place between the individual who is desiring to have the HRPF assessment and the professional who will be administering the assessments. It is through the process of articulating the purposes, risks, and benefits of the assessment that professionals help their clients have the knowledge and understanding needed to make informed decisions about whether to complete the HRPF assessment. Although the evidence suggests that for most people expected benefits of performing the assessment outweigh the associated risks, each client needs to make an informed decision based on personal factors.

BOX 2.1	**Sample of Informed Consent Form for a Symptom-Limited Exercise Test**

Informed Consent for an Exercise Test

1. Purpose and Explanation of the Test

You will perform an exercise test on a cycle ergometer or a motor-driven treadmill. The exercise intensity will begin at a low level and will be advanced in stages depending on your fitness level. We may stop the test at any time because of signs of fatigue or changes in your heart rate, electrocardiogram, or blood pressure, or symptoms you may experience. It is important for you to realize that you may stop when you wish because of feelings of fatigue or any other discomfort.

2. Attendant Risks and Discomforts

There exists the possibility of certain changes occurring during the test. These include abnormal blood pressure; fainting; irregular, fast, or slow heart rhythm; and, in rare instances, heart attack, stroke, or death. Every effort will be made to minimize these risks by evaluation of preliminary information relating to your health and fitness and by careful observations during testing. Emergency equipment and trained personnel are available to deal with unusual situations that may arise.

3. Responsibilities of the Participant

Information you possess about your health status or previous experiences of heart-related symptoms (*e.g.*, shortness of breath with low-level activity; pain; pressure; tightness; heaviness in the chest, neck, jaw, back, and/or arms) with physical effort may affect the safety of your exercise test. Your prompt reporting of these and any other unusual feelings with effort during the exercise test itself is very important. You are responsible for fully disclosing your medical history as well as symptoms that may occur during the test. You are also expected to report all medications (including nonprescription) taken recently and, in particular, those taken today to the testing staff.

4. Benefits To Be Expected

The results obtained from the exercise test may assist in the diagnosis of your illness, in evaluating the effect of your medications, or in evaluating what type of physical activities you might do with low risk.

5. Inquiries

Any questions about the procedures used in the exercise test or the results of your test are encouraged. If you have any concerns or questions, please ask us for further explanations.

6. Use of Medical Records

The information that is obtained during exercise testing will be treated as privileged and confidential as described in the Health Insurance Portability and Accountability Act of 1996. It is not to be released or revealed to any individual except your referring physician without your written consent. However, the information obtained may be used for statistical analysis or scientific purposes with your right to privacy retained.

7. Freedom of Consent

I hereby consent to voluntarily engage in an exercise test to determine my exercise capacity and state of cardiovascular health. My permission to perform this exercise test is given voluntarily. I understand that I am free to stop the test at any point if I so desire.

I have read this form, and I understand the test procedures that I will perform and the attendant risks and discomforts. Knowing these risks and discomforts, and having had an opportunity to ask questions that have been answered to my satisfaction, I consent to participate in this test.

Date	Signature of Patient
Date	Signature of Witness
Date	Signature of Physician or Authorized Delegate

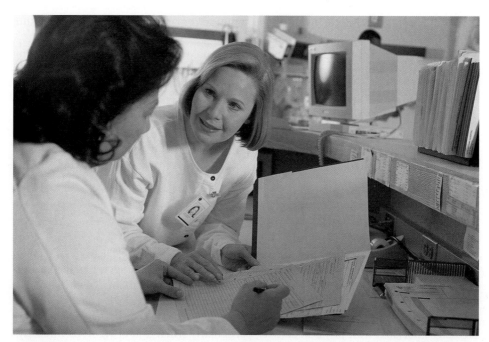

■ **FIGURE 2.1.** An important aspect of the informed consent process is reviewing key elements with the client and answering any questions the client may have.

To begin the informed consent process, the client should carefully read the entire form or have the form read aloud while following along. Next, the professional should review some of the key elements of the assessment including purpose, risks and benefits, and overview of procedures (*Fig. 2.1*). One key point of emphasis is that the client will play an important role in the process. Specifically, the client has the responsibility of informing test administrators of any problems experienced (past, present, and during the physical fitness assessment) that may increase the risk of the test or preclude participation. This information is essential to minimize the risks involved with the assessment and can also optimize the benefits. Finally, the client should be allowed and encouraged to ask any questions before completing the informed consent process with a signature.

EXPLANATION OF PROCEDURES

The professional should be prepared to provide a brief description of each assessment to be performed and answer client questions in detail. The following are examples of some common HRPF assessments and sample explanations of each. A more detailed review of all the HRPF assessments is provided in *Chapters 4–8*.

- Anthropometry or body composition: "This test is being performed to obtain an estimate of your total body fat percentage. We will determine your body fat percentage by taking measurements with a set of calipers at different sites on your body. We do this by pinching and pulling on the skin at these different locations. We will also measure some body girths with a tape measure to provide an indication of distribution of the fat on your body."
- Cardiorespiratory fitness: "This test is being performed to obtain an estimate of your cardiorespiratory fitness. The test will require you to exercise on a stationary cycle for 6–12 min. The intensity of the test will be limited to a level below your maximal

exertion point. During the test, we will monitor your heart rate and blood pressure response to the submaximal exercise."

- Flexibility: "While there is no one test of your total range of motion, this test is being performed to obtain a measure of the flexibility of your lower back and legs. We will measure how far you can reach, to or beyond your toes, while sitting with your legs straight."
- Muscular fitness: "While there is no one test that can measure your total muscular fitness, this test is being performed to obtain a measure of your muscle strength by having you squeeze a hand grip dynamometer as hard as you can. We will also measure muscle endurance by having you perform as many sit-ups as you can in a 1-min time period."

SCREENING PROCEDURES

Preassessment screening is the next step in the process of HRPF assessment. Preassessment screening is a process of gathering a client's demographic and health-related information along with some health risk/medical assessments (see *Chapter 3*). This information may be used for determining the individual's risks for chronic disease and risks related to physical activity participation. As noted earlier in this chapter, there are risks associated with physical activity, particularly when it is of vigorous intensity.

Chapter 2 of the *ACSM's GETP9* provides a thorough overview of what is termed preparticipation health screening process. Although very similar to the preassessment screening, preparticipation screening procedures are designed principally to provide guidance for previously inactive individuals who wish to initiate a regular exercise program or for those who perform moderate or irregular exercise but desire to increase the vigor and regularity of their exercise. ACSM "supports the public health message that all people should adopt a physically active lifestyle" and believes that the preparticipation health screening process should not include "unnecessary and unproven barriers to adopting a physically active lifestyle." Indeed, the *2008 Physical Activity Guidelines for Americans* provided the following guidance:

> *The protective value of a medical consultation for persons with or without chronic diseases who are interested in increasing their physical activity level is not established. People without diagnosed chronic conditions (such as diabetes, heart disease, or osteoarthritis) and who do not have symptoms (such as chest pain or pressure, dizziness, or joint pain) do not need to consult a health-care provider about physical activity (9).*

Whereas preparticipation screening is typically incorporated for the person beginning an exercise program, preassessment screening is employed for the person wanting to perform a comprehensive HRPF assessment. Although the decision-making process in these two situations may be similar, there are key differences between the two with respect to risk. As stated earlier, physical activity-related risks are influenced by both the intensity of the activity and the activity habits of the client. Some HRPF assessments require vigorous-to-maximal intensity exercise, and it is not uncommon to perform these measures on clients who have not been regularly active. In these circumstances, the preassessment health screening process may need to be more involved.

The preassessment screening, like the informed consent, is a dynamic process. It may vary in its scope and components depending on the client's needs based on health and medical status (*e.g.*, health conditions or diseases), the type of HRPF assessments gathered (*e.g.*, submaximal vs. maximal cardiorespiratory fitness tests), and the physical activity or exercise program goals (*e.g.*, moderate intensity vs. vigorous intensity).

There are many reasons why clients should be screened prior to involvement in an HRPF assessment program. These include the following:

- To identify those with a medical contraindication (exclusion), as outlined in *Box 2.2*, to performing specific HRPF assessments
- To identify those who should receive a medical evaluation conducted by a physician prior to performing specific HRPF assessments
- To identify those who should only perform some specific (vigorous) HRPF assessments administered by professionals with clinical experience (and possibly in a clinical facility with physician availability)
- To identify those with other health risk/medical concerns (*e.g.*, diabetes mellitus or orthopedic injuries) that may influence the decision about performing specific HRPF assessments or the need to modify assessment procedures

---

BOX 2.2   Contraindications to Exercise Testing

ABSOLUTE
- A recent significant change in the resting electrocardiogram (ECG) suggesting significant ischemia, recent myocardial infarction (within 2 d), or other acute cardiac event
- Unstable angina
- Uncontrolled cardiac dysrhythmias causing symptoms or hemodynamic compromise
- Symptomatic severe aortic stenosis
- Uncontrolled symptomatic heart failure
- Acute pulmonary embolus or pulmonary infarction
- Acute myocarditis or pericarditis
- Suspected or known dissecting aneurysm
- Acute systemic infection, accompanied by fever, body aches, or swollen lymph glands

RELATIVE[a]
- Left main coronary stenosis
- Moderate stenotic valvular heart disease
- Electrolyte abnormalities (*e.g.*, hypokalemia or hypomagnesemia)
- Severe arterial hypertension (*i.e.*, systolic blood pressure [SBP] of >200 mm Hg and/or a diastolic BP [DBP] of >110 mm Hg) at rest
- Tachydysrhythmia or bradydysrhythmia
- Hypertrophic cardiomyopathy and other forms of outflow tract obstruction
- Neuromotor, musculoskeletal, or rheumatoid disorders that are exacerbated by exercise
- High-degree atrioventricular block
- Ventricular aneurysm
- Uncontrolled metabolic disease (*e.g.*, diabetes, thyrotoxicosis, or myxedema)
- Chronic infectious disease (*e.g.*, HIV)
- Mental or physical impairment leading to inability to exercise adequately

[a]Relative contraindications can be superseded if benefits outweigh the risks of exercise. In some instances, these individuals can be exercised with caution and/or using low-level endpoints, especially if they are asymptomatic at rest.
Modified from (4) cited 2007 June 15. Available from: http://www.ncbi.nlm.nih.gov/pubmed/12356646

HEALTH HISTORY QUESTIONNAIRE

Most of the pertinent health risks and medical information about a client can be obtained from a health history questionnaire (HHQ). A well-designed HHQ should note the individual's current activity habits; identify any serious medical conditions (contraindications to exercise); document any known cardiovascular, pulmonary, or renal diseases or the presence of diabetes; and determine cardiovascular disease risk factors. The HHQ can be tailored to fit the specific information required of the type of HRPF assessment being performed. For example, little health risk and medical information is needed if the client is only performing a body composition assessment. However, clients interested in performing assessments requiring maximal exercise should complete a comprehensive HHQ. In general, the HHQ should assess a client's

- cardiovascular disease risk factors,
- past history and present status of any signs and symptoms suggestive of cardiovascular disease,
- history of chronic diseases and illnesses,
- history of surgeries and hospitalizations,
- history of any musculoskeletal and joint injuries,
- past and present health behaviors/habits (physical activity, dietary patterns, weight loss), and
- current use of any medications.

An example of a comprehensive health history form is shown in *Figure* 2.2.

Contraindications for Exercise

It is critically important to recognize that a client may have medical conditions for which exercise should not be performed until the condition is resolved. These are conditions for which the immediate risks of exercise outweigh any potential benefit that could be derived from the exercise. These are called contraindications for exercise and are listed in *Box* 2.2. Clients identified with these factors should not perform an HRPF assessment and should be informed to seek medical attention for the condition.

Cardiovascular Disease Risk Factors

The cardiovascular disease risk factors' thresholds used in the American College of Sports Medicine (ACSM) risk classification process are listed in *Table 2.1*. To determine levels of risk, the ACSM uses criteria established by other professional organizations such as the National Cholesterol Education Program (NCEP). However, slightly different risk factor criteria may be found in some other sources.

It is important to follow the specific criteria for determining the presence or absence of the cardiovascular disease risk factors. For example, note that age thresholds differ between the age risk factor and the family history risk factor. Also, for the blood pressure and hyperlipidemia risk factors, repeat assessments are necessary to confirm the measurement. Further, those whose conditions are controlled by medications are still considered to have the risk factors.

The low and moderate risk classification of a client is determined by the numerical total of all risk factors. Note that there are eight positive risk factors and one negative risk factor used by ACSM for risk classification. If a client has high high-density lipoprotein (HDL) cholesterol, then 1 is subtracted from the sum of the positive risk factors to determine the total number of risk factors for risk stratification.

TODAY'S DATE _____

NAME _____ AGE _____ DATE OF BIRTH _____

ADDRESS _____
    Street   City   State   Zip

TELEPHONE: HOME/CELL _____/ _____ E-MAIL ADDRESS _____

OCCUPATION/EMPLOYER _____/ _____ BUSINESS PHONE _____

MARITAL STATUS: (check one) SINGLE ☐   MARRIED ☐   DIVORCED ☐   WIDOWED ☐

PERSONAL PHYSICIAN _____ PHONE # _____

ADDRESS _____

Reason for last doctor visit?_____ Date of last physical exam: _____

Have you ever had any other exercise stress test?   YES ☐   NO ☐   DATE & LOCATION OF TEST: _____
_____

Have you ever had any cardiovascular tests?   YES ☐   NO ☐   DATE & LOCATION: _____
_____

Person to contact in case of an emergency _____ Phone _____ (relationship) _____

Please provide responses (YES or NO) to the following concerning family history, your own history, and any symptoms you have had:

FAMILY HISTORY		
Have any immediate family members had a:	YES	NO
heart attack	o	o
heart surgery	o	o
coronary stent	o	o
cardiac catheterization	o	o
congenital heart defect	o	o
stroke	o	o
Other chronic disease: _____		
_____		
_____		
_____		
_____		

PERSONAL HISTORY		
Have you ever had:	YES	NO
High blood pressure	o	o
High cholesterol	o	o
Diabetes	o	o
Any heart problems	o	o
Disease of arteries	o	o
Thyroid disease	o	o
Lung disease	o	o
Asthma	o	o
Cancer	o	o
Kidney disease	o	o
Hepatitis	o	o
Other: _____		

SYMPTOMS		
Have you ever had:	YES	NO
Chest pain	o	o
Shortness of breath	o	o
Heart palpitations	o	o
Skipped heartbeats	o	o
Heart murmur	o	o
Intermittent leg pain	o	o
Dizziness or fainting	o	o
Fatigue — usual activities	o	o
Snoring	o	o
Back pain	o	o
Orthopedic problems	o	o
Other: _____		

STAFF COMMENTS: _____
_____
_____

Have you ever had your cholesterol measured?   Yes ☐   No ☐   If yes, value _____ Where: _____

Are you taking any prescription (include birth control pills) or nonprescription medications?   Yes ☐   No ☐
For each of your current medications, provide the following information:

MEDICATION   Dosage—times/day   Time taken   Years on medication   Reason for taking
_____
_____
_____

HOSPITALIZATIONS: Please list recent hospitalizations (Women: do not list normal pregnancies)

■ **FIGURE 2.2.** An example of a comprehensive health history questionnaire (HHQ). Source: Ball State University — Clinical Exercise Physiology Program.

Year	Location	Reason

_____

_____

_____

Any other medical problems/concerns not already identified?   Yes ☐   No ☐   If so, please list: _____

_____

_____

LIFESTYLE HABITS

Do you ever have an uncomfortable shortness of breath during exercise or when doing activities?

   Yes ☐   No ☐

Do you ever have chest discomfort during exercise?   Yes ☐   No ☐

   If so, does it go away with rest?   Yes ☐   No ☐

_____

Do you currently smoke?   Yes ☐   No ☐   If so, what? Cigarettes ☐   Cigars ☐   Pipe ☐

   How long have you smoked? _____ years

How much per day: <½ pack ☐   ½ to 1 pack ☐   1 to 1½ packs ☐   1½ to 2 packs ☐   >2 packs ☐

Have you ever quit smoking?   Yes ☐   No ☐   When? _____

   How many years and how much did you smoke? _____

Do you drink any alcoholic beverages?   Yes ☐   No ☐   If yes, how much in 1 week? (indicate below)

   Beer _____ (cans)   Wine _____ (glasses)   Hard liquor _____ (drinks)

Do you drink any caffeinated beverages?   Yes ☐   No ☐   If yes, how much in 1 week? (indicate below)

   Coffee _____ (cups)   Tea _____ (glasses)   Soft drinks _____ (cans)

Are you currently following a weight reduction diet plan?   Yes ☐   No ☐

   If so, how long have you been dieting? _____ months

   Is the plan prescribed by your doctor?   Yes ☐   No ☐

Have you used weight reduction diets in the past?   Yes ☐   No ☐   If yes, how often and what type? ____

_____

ACTIVITY LEVEL EVALUATION

What is your occupational activity level?   Sedentary ☐   Light ☐   Moderate ☐   Heavy ☐

Do you currently engage in vigorous physical activity on a regular basis?   Yes ☐   No ☐

   If so, what type(s)? _____ How many days per week? _____

   How much time per day?   <15 min ☐   15–30 min ☐   31–60 min ☐   >60 min ☐

   How long have you engaged in this type of activity?   <3 months ☐   3–12 months ☐   >1 year ☐

_____

Do you engage in any recreational or leisure-time physical activities on a regular basis?   Yes ☐   No ☐

   If so, what activities? _____

   On average: How often? _____ times/week;   for how long? _____ time/session

   How long have you engaged in this type of activity?   <3 months   3–12 months   >1 year

_____

Your fitness goals and objectives are: _____

_____

STAFF COMMENTS: _____

_____

_____

■ **FIGURE 2.2.** _Continued._

TABLE 2.1. Atherosclerotic Cardiovascular Disease (CVD) Risk Factors and Defining Criteria (8,12)

Risk Factors	Defining Criteria
Age	Men ≥45 yr; women ≥55 yr (4)
Family history	Myocardial infarction, coronary revascularization, or sudden death before 55 yr in father or other male first-degree relative or before 65 yr in mother or other female first-degree relative
Cigarette smoking	Current cigarette smoker or those who quit within the previous 6 mo or exposure to environmental tobacco smoke
Sedentary lifestyle	Not participating in at least 30 min of moderate intensity, physical activity (40%–<60% $\dot{V}O_2R$) on at least 3 d of the week for at least 3 mo (7,10)
Obesity	Body mass index ≥30 kg · m⁻² *or* waist girth >102 cm (40 in) for men and >88 cm (35 in) for women (3)
Hypertension	Systolic blood pressure ≥140 mm Hg and/or diastolic ≥90 mm Hg, confirmed by measurements on at least two separate occasions, *or* on antihypertensive medication (2)
Dyslipidemia	Low-density lipoprotein (LDL) cholesterol ≥130 mg · dL⁻¹ (3.37 mmol · L⁻¹) *or* high-density lipoprotein[b] (HDL) cholesterol <40 mg · dL⁻¹ (1.04 mmol · L⁻¹) *or* on lipid-lowering medication. If total serum cholesterol is all that is available, use ≥200 mg · dL⁻¹ (5.18 mmol · L⁻¹) (6)
Prediabetes[a]	Impaired fasting glucose (IFG) = fasting plasma glucose ≥100 mg · dL⁻¹ (5.55 mmol · L⁻¹) and ≤125 mg · dL⁻¹ (6.94 mmol · L⁻¹) or impaired glucose tolerance (IGT) = 2 h values in oral glucose tolerance test (OGTT) ≥140 mg · dL⁻¹ (7.77 mmol · L⁻¹) and ≤199 mg · dL⁻¹ (11.04 mmol · L⁻¹) confirmed by measurements on at least two separate occasions (1)
Negative Risk Factors	**Defining Criteria**
High-density lipoprotein (HDL) cholesterol	≥60 mg · dL⁻¹ (1.55 mmol · L⁻¹)

[a]If the presence or absence of a CVD risk factor is not disclosed or is not available, that CVD risk factor should be counted as a risk factor except for prediabetes. If the prediabetes criteria are missing or unknown, prediabetes should be counted as a risk factor for those ≥45 yr, especially for those with a body mass index (BMI) ≥25 kg · m⁻², and those <45 yr with a BMI ≥25 kg · m⁻² and additional CVD risk factors for prediabetes. The number of positive risk factors is then summed.

[b]High HDL is considered a negative risk factor. For individuals having high HDL ≥60 mg · dL⁻¹ (1.55 mmol · L⁻¹), for these individuals one positive risk factor is subtracted from the sum of positive risk factors.

$\dot{V}O_2R$, oxygen uptake reserve.

Signs or Symptoms Suggestive of Cardiopulmonary Disease

There are several visible signs or reported symptoms a client may have that would indicate the likelihood of having a cardiovascular, pulmonary, or metabolic disease. These signs and symptoms are listed in *Table 2.2*. If a client has any of these signs or symptoms, then the client is placed in the high-risk classification, regardless of the presence or absence of any cardiovascular disease risk factors. A client with a sign or symptom should be immediately referred to a physician for follow-up and to obtain medical clearance prior to participation in the assessments.

To make a decision about the presence or absence of a sign or symptom suggestive of cardiovascular, pulmonary, or metabolic disease, be sure to follow the specific criteria. Some key features that aid in clarifying whether the reported feeling should be designated as a symptom are listed in *Table 2.2*. For example, a client may report that he or she has experienced chest pain. The key features that classify this pain as *favoring an ischemic origin* are the *character* of the pain, the *location* of the pain, and the

TABLE 2.2. Major Signs or Symptoms Suggestive of Cardiovascular, Pulmonary, or Metabolic Disease

Pain, discomfort in the chest, neck, jaw, arms, or other areas that may result from ischemia

Shortness of breath at rest or with mild exertion

Dizziness or syncope

Orthopnea or paroxysmal nocturnal dyspnea

Ankle edema

Palpitations or tachycardia

Intermittent claudication

Known heart murmur

Unusual fatigue or shortness of breath with usual activities

For more explanation of these signs and symptoms see *GETP9 Table 2.1.*

factors associated with *provoking* the pain. It is important to ask the client to describe the feeling with as little prompting for specific characteristics as possible. Ideally, you want the client to describe the feeling using self-selected words. Asking a client to describe the location of the pain is better than asking if there is pain in the shoulders, neck, or arms.

Recommendations Following Screening

ACSM recommends classifying individuals into one of three levels of risk according to the criteria presented in *Table 2.3*. The logic involved in determining the correct classification is depicted in *Figure 2.3*. The risk classification determined then dictates the appropriate course of action regarding participation in moderate or vigorous intensity exercise, which is certainly involved in many fitness assessments. This approach, as presented in *Figure 2.4*, begins with decisions about the recommendation to have a medical exam and also includes recommendations for the level of training that is appropriate for supervision of both submaximal and maximal exercise tests. It is important to point out that as stated in *ACSM's GETP9* "a periodic health examination or a similar contact with a health care provider should be encouraged as part of routine health maintenance and to detect medical conditions unrelated to exercise."

The first decision to be made is to determine if the client should be advised to have a medical exam prior to participation in activities (including HRPF assessments) that require moderate or vigorous intensity. Regardless of the intensity of the exercise, clients

TABLE 2.3. ACSM Risk Classification Categories

Low risk	Asymptomatic men and women who have <2 CVD risk factor from *Table 2.1*
Moderate risk	Asymptomatic men and women who have ≥2 risk factors from *Table 2.1*
High risk	Individuals who have any signs and symptoms listed in *Table 2.2* or have a known cardiovascular,[a] pulmonary,[b] or renal disease or diabetes

[a]Cardiac, peripheral vascular, or cerebrovascular disease.
[b]Chronic obstructive pulmonary disease, asthma, interstitial lung disease, or cystic fibrosis.
ACSM, American College of Sports Medicine; CVD, cardiovascular disease.

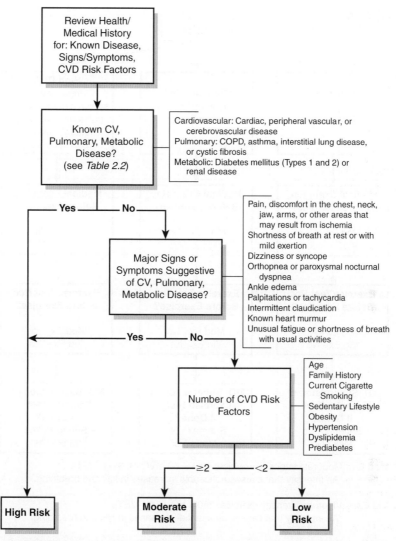

■ **FIGURE 2.3.** Logic model for classification of risk. CV, cardiovascular; CVD, cardio-vascular disease.

classified as high risk are advised to have a medical examination, and those with a low risk receive no such recommendation. The recommendation for clients in the moderate risk classification depends on the intensity of exercise. No medical examination need precede the performance of moderate intensity activities or assessments, although such an exam is recommended prior to the performance of vigorous intensity activities or assessments. These recommendations are consistent with those from the *2008 Physical Activity Guidelines for Americans*, which stated:

> *Health-care providers can provide useful personalized advice on how to reduce risk of injuries. For people who wish to seek the advice of a health-care provider, it is particularly appropriate to do so when contemplating vigorous-intensity activity, because the risks of this activity are higher than the risks of moderate-intensity activity (9).*

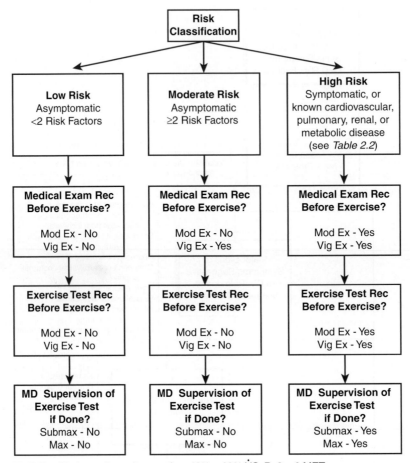

Mod Ex: Moderate intensity exercise; 40%–<60% $\dot{V}O_2R$; 3–<6 METs
"An intensity that causes noticeable increases in HR and breathing."

Vig Ex: Vigorous intensity exercise; ≥60% $\dot{V}O_2R$; ≥6 METs
"An intensity that causes substantial increases in HR and breathing."

Not Rec: Reflects the notion a medical examination, exercise test, and physician supervision of exercise testing are not recommended in the preparticipation screening; however, they may be considered when there are concerns about risk, more information is needed for the Ex R_x, and/or are requested by the patient or client.

Rec: Reflects the notion a medical examination, exercise test, and physician supervision are recommended in the preparticipation health screening process.

■ **FIGURE 2.4.** Medical examination, exercise testing, and supervision of exercise testing preparticipation recommendations based on classification of risk. Ex R_x, exercise prescription; HR, heart rate; METs, metabolic equivalents; $\dot{V}O_2R$, oxygen uptake reserve.

Fitness professionals should always use prudent judgment when deciding whether a client needs a medical examination prior to HRPF assessment. If unsure, select the conservative option and require a physician's clearance.

Once a determination is made to proceed with the exercise-based assessment, then a second decision relating to the recommendation of an exercise test, and if done, the training level of the staff administering submaximal or maximal exercise tests must be made. ACSM does not consider it necessary to recommend an exercise test for clients in the low and moderate risk classifications. However, if an exercise test is elected and performed by low- and moderate-risk clients, then ACSM does not consider it necessary to recommend physician supervision. For all clients classified as high risk, an exercise test is recommended prior to participation in moderate-to-vigorous assessments, and physician supervision is recommended for either submaximal or maximal exercise tests. It is important to understand that this process is only a recommended guide for action as described in *ACSM's GETP9*: "No set of guidelines for exercise testing prior to initiation of physical activity covers all situations. Local circumstances and policies vary, and specific program procedures are also properly diverse."

OTHER HEALTH ISSUES TO CONSIDER

Note that the ACSM and American Heart Association (AHA) screening recommendations are focused mostly on cardiovascular risk issues (5). If the screening identifies a medical history of musculoskeletal problems, then a similar referral to a health care provider should be made before any HRPF assessments that could impact the musculoskeletal condition.

UNDERSTANDING MEDICATION USAGE

A list of all medications that a client is presently using should be obtained during the preassessment screening. It is beyond the level of expertise for a nonclinical exercise professional to have a complete understanding of all medications. However, the fitness professional should minimally know if a client is taking any medications and whether the medication may alter the client's response to acute or chronic exercise. There are many sources to review medications, their side effects, and how they impact the exercise response. Some sources are quite detailed and are beyond the scope of information needed by the fitness professional. The U.S. National Library of Medicine and the National Institutes of Health provide a straightforward Web site, which allows for a search of a specific medication and yields information regarding usage, side effects, and precautions (11). Additionally, *ACSM's GETP9* provides information on medications in *Appendix A*.

The fitness professional should not instruct a client to stop taking or change the timing of his or her medication prior to any HRPF assessment. Only the client's physician should make such decisions.

SUMMARY

Preassessment screening includes informed consent, risk classification, and determination of the recommendations for a medical evaluation prior to performing the HRPF assessment. The informed consent is a process that involves several key elements, allowing the client to completely understand the essential factors related to performing the HRPF assessment. The risk classification helps the fitness professional guide the client in making decisions about health readiness to proceed with the HRPF assessment. Depending on the client's risk level, a referral to the client's health care provider may be important prior to proceeding with the assessment.

LABORATORY ACTIVITIES

RISK CLASSIFICATION USING A COMPREHENSIVE HEALTH HISTORY QUESTIONNAIRE

Data Collection

Ask a friend or relative older than the age of 45 yr to complete the comprehensive HHQ (be sure to omit a name or any identifying information with your assignment). Review the questionnaire with this individual.

Written Report

Determine this person's ACSM risk classification. Provide the criteria for the selection of the correct ACSM risk classification.

EVALUATION OF MEDICATIONS PRIOR TO PARTICIPATION IN A PHYSICAL FITNESS EVALUTION

Data Collection

Ask a friend or relative older than the age of 55 yr that is presently taking three or more medications to provide you with a complete list of the names of each medication along with the dosage and frequency of use (be sure to omit a name or any identifying information with your assignment).

Written Report

Provide a summary of the following for each medication:

- The reason the person is taking the medication (*i.e.*, the indication for use)
- The common side effects of the medication
- The potential for this medication effecting the person's response to exercise; especially note if the medication may change the person's heart rate

ADMINISTERING AN INFORMED CONSENT

In-Class Project

With a laboratory partner, practice verbally reviewing the key elements of an informed consent and providing an explanation of procedures for a body composition assessment.

CASE STUDY

Todd is a 44-yr-old electrical engineer who works 50–60 h · wk^{-1}. He is 5 ft. 9 in, 233 lb, with total cholesterol of 192 mg · dL^{-1}, low-density lipoprotein (LDL) of 138 mg · dL^{-1}, HDL of 41 mg · dL^{-1}, triglycerides of 200 mg · dL^{-1}, and blood glucose of 120 mg · dL^{-1}. Todd's resting heart rate is 81 beats per minute (bpm) and blood pressure is 144/86 mm Hg. His waist and hip circumference measures are 42 in and 40 in, respectively. Todd has never smoked but usually has one to two glasses of wine with dinner. He reports no leisure-time physical activity and does not exercise on a regular basis (less than two sessions per month). Todd denies all complaints of chest discomfort and shortness of breath at rest or with exertion;

Case Study, cont.

however, he has gained 20 lb over the last 2 yr. Todd's wife reports he snores frequently and has difficulty waking up in the mornings. Further testing reveals that Todd has obstructive sleep apnea and is being treated with continuous positive airway pressure (CPAP). A review of his family history reveals that Todd's father had double bypass surgery at the age of 53 and suffered a fatal myocardial infarction at the age of 62. Todd's brother (42 yr old) also is hypertensive and was recently diagnosed with Type 2 diabetes, which is being treated with diet and physical activity recommendations. Todd has been referred to your facility for coronary artery disease risk factor reduction and physical activity counseling.

Determine the presence or absence of each CVD risk factor, any signs or symptoms, the ACSM risk classification, the recommendations for a medical exam and exercise test, and the use of physician supervision of the exercise test.

REFERENCES

1. American Diabetes Association. Diagnosis and classification of diabetes mellitus. *Diabetes Care*. 2007; 30(suppl 1):S42–7.
2. Chobanian AV, Bakris GL, Black HR, et al. The seventh report of the Joint National Committee on Prevention, Detection, Evaluation, and Treatment of High Blood Pressure: the JNC 7 report. *JAMA*. 2003; 289(19):2560–72.
3. Executive summary of the clinical guidelines on the identification, evaluation, and treatment of overweight and obesity in adults. *Arch Intern Med*. 1998;158(17):1855–67.
4. Gibbons RJ, Balady GJ, Bricker JT, et al. ACC/AHA 2002 guideline update for exercise testing: summary article. A report of the American College of Cardiology/American Heart Association Task Force on Practice Guidelines (Committee to Update the 1997 Exercise Testing Guidelines). *J Am Coll Cardiol*. 2002;40(8):1531–40.
5. Lloyd-Jones DM, Hong Y, Labarthe D, et al. Defining and setting national goals for cardiovascular health promotion and disease reduction: the American Heart Association's Strategic Impact Goal through 2020 and beyond. *Circulation*. 2010;121:586–613.
6. National Cholesterol Education Program Expert Panel on Detection, Evaluation, and Treatment of High Blood Cholesterol in Adults (Adult Treatment Panel III). Third Report of the National Cholesterol Education Program (NCEP) Expert Panel on Detection, Evaluation, and Treatment of High Blood Cholesterol in Adults (Adult Treatment Panel III) final report. *Circulation*. 2002;106(25):3143–421.
7. Pate RR, Pratt M, Blair SN, et al. Physical activity and public health. A recommendation from the Centers for Disease Control and Prevention and the American College of Sports Medicine. *JAMA*. 1995;273(5): 402–7.
8. Roger VL, Go AS, Lloyd-Jones DM, et al. Heart Disease and Stroke Statistics—2012 Update: a report from the American Heart Association. *Circulation*. 2012;125(1):e2–220.
9. U.S. Department of Health and Human Services. *2008 Physical Activity Guidelines for Americans*. ODPHP publication U0036 [Internet]. 2008 [cited 2011 Jul 10]. Available from: www.health.gov/paguidelines
10. U.S. Department of Human Health and Services. *Physical Activity and Health: A Report of the Surgeon General*. Atlanta, GA: U.S. Department of Health and Human Services, Centers for Disease Control and Prevention, National Center for Chronic Disease Prevention and Health Promotion; 1996. 278 p.
11. U.S. National Library of Medicine and National Institutes of Health. *Medline Plus: Drugs, supplements and Herbal Information* [Internet]. 2011 [cited 2011 Jul 11]. Available from: www.nlm.nih.gov/medlineplus/druginformation.html
12. U.S. Preventive Services Task Force. Screening for coronary heart disease: recommendation statement. *Ann Intern Med*. 2004;140(7):569–72.

3

Risk Factor Assessments

RATIONALE FOR RISK ASSESSMENT

The importance of risk assessment was discussed in *Chapter 2*. A client who is an active participant in his or her health care will likely have many risk factors measured and monitored through regular medical checkups. These individuals can provide most of the necessary risk assessment information via self-report on a health history questionnaire. However, many clients may not regularly see a physician or may not have had these measurements taken for over a year. Thus, an important service for personnel who provide health-related physical fitness (HRPF) assessments is to also provide measurements of common risk factors and screenings for other chronic diseases. Additionally, these measures may stimulate a client to pay more attention to their personal health when risk factors are detected, motivating them to make positive health-related changes. In some cases, results may even identify individuals who need to seek medical follow-up.

RESTING BLOOD PRESSURE

Blood pressure (BP) is the force of blood against the walls of the arteries and veins created by the heart as it pumps blood to every part of the body. For a health risk assessment, arterial BP is measured and expressed in units of millimeters of mercury (mm Hg). Two phases of BP, systolic and diastolic, are assessed. The systolic BP (SBP) is the maximum pressure in the arteries during the contraction (systole) phase of the heart. Diastolic BP (DBP) is the minimum pressure in the arteries during the relaxation (diastole) phase of the heart. BP measurements are used in risk classification, as was discussed in *Chapter 2* (see *Fig. 2.3*).

MEASUREMENT

The direct measure of BP requires placement of a catheter in an artery followed by the insertion of a pressure transducer into the catheter. Obviously, this is an invasive procedure that can only be performed by trained clinical professionals. Although often used during surgical operations and within research settings, the direct method is not required for determining resting BP in routine health care practice. Resting BP is typically assessed by employing an indirect method termed auscultation. Auscultation involves listening to internal sounds of the body using a stethoscope. For BP assessment, a stethoscope is placed over an artery to listen for the sounds of Korotkoff on the arterial walls. The five phases of the Korotkoff sounds are provided in *Box 3.1*. The sounds of Korotkoff heard through the stethoscope during the BP measurement come from the turbulence of blood in the artery, which is caused by blood moving from an area of higher pressure to an area of lower pressure. A cuff is applied to the upper arm

---

BOX 3.1 Korotkoff Sounds

- Phase 1. The first, initial sound or the onset of sound. Sounds like clear, repetitive tapping. The sound may be faint at first and gradually increase in intensity or volume to phase 2.
- Phase 2. Sounds like a soft tapping or murmur. The sounds are often longer than the phase 1 sounds. These sounds have also been described as having a swishing component. The phase 2 sounds are typically 10–15 mm Hg after the onset of sound (phase 1).
- Phase 3. Sounds like a loud tapping sound; high in both pitch and intensity. These sounds are crisper and louder than the phase 2 sounds.
- Phase 4. Sounds like a muffling of the sound. The sounds become less distinct and less audible. Another way of describing this sound is as soft or blowing.
- Phase 5. Sounds like the complete disappearance of sound. The true disappearance of sound usually occurs within 8–10 mm Hg of the muffling of sound (phase 4).

and is inflated with air by pumping up a hand bulb. This air pressure inside the BP cuff occludes the blood flow within the brachial artery. As long as the pressure in the cuff is higher than the SBP, the artery remains occluded or collapsed and no sound is heard through the applied stethoscope. When the air pressure is slowly released from the cuff, the pressure inside the cuff will eventually equal the driving pressure of the blood in the artery and the first sound will be heard in the stethoscope. This sound corresponds to the measure of SBP. As the pressure in the cuff continues to drop, it will eventually get to a point where the cuff is no longer occluding the artery and all sounds will disappear. The pressure reading at the last sound heard is the DBP.

Measurement Equipment

BP measurement using the auscultatory method requires a stethoscope, a manometer or sphygmomanometer (a device to measure pressure), and a cuff with an inflatable bladder that is wrapped around the limb (typically the arm). The two common types of manometers used for BP measurement are mercury and aneroid as shown in *Figure 3.1*. Mercury, the standard for pressure measurements, is housed in a small reservoir (~300 mm) located at the base of a vertical glass column. However, because mercury is a toxic chemical, aneroid sphygmomanometers are becoming more common in the workplace. Indeed, many facilities have instituted a ban on all devices containing mercury. Further, regulations for disposal of mercury must be followed and vary by state. Knowledge of

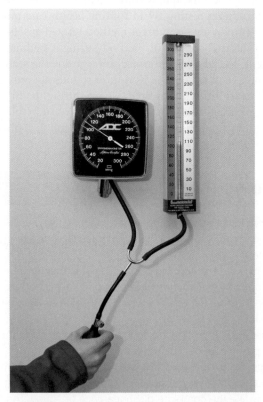

■ **FIGURE 3.1.** A Y tube is used to perform a calibration check of aneroid manometers. (Photograph by Ball State University.)

state and facility regulations regarding mercury use and disposal is imperative and can be researched through the U.S. Environmental Protection Agency (27).

Aneroid sphygmomanometers measure the pressure in the cuff by the movement of a spring-loaded needle that moves on a dial-type scale. Facilities should have at least three different BP cuff sizes available: small, medium, and large. There are index lines on many of the newer sphygmomanometer cuffs to help determine the correct cuff for a client's arm circumference. Typically, the appropriate BP bladder (the inflatable rubber sac within the cuff) should encircle at least 80% of the arm's circumference without overlapping. In general, a bladder within the cuff that is too small will result in an overestimation of BP and a cuff that is too long will result in an underestimation of BP.

Equipment used in the measurement of BP is widely available commercially but varies greatly in quality. Sphygmomanometer units can be purchased in most pharmacies, various health and fitness commercial catalogs, and medical supply stores. A high-quality stethoscope is worth the investment to help in hearing clear Korotkoff sounds.

Automated Systems

Electronic BP machines have been available for many years, and industrial models are increasingly being used in both hospitals and doctors' offices. Commercial models have also become relatively inexpensive for individuals who wish to self-monitor BP at home (19). Most of these systems use the oscillatory method for measuring BP. This method uses a cuff that fills with a fluid instead of air. SBP is detected when oscillations begin during the deflation of the pressure, with DBP being recorded at the point of maximal oscillations. Although these devices have been shown to provide reasonably accurate BP measurements, they are limited by the lack of a simple and inexpensive method to verify their calibration over time.

Calibration of an Aneroid Manometer

The aneroid manometer needs to be checked regularly for accuracy against the standard mercury manometer. Because this calibration check procedure requires only a few minutes, it is reasonable to suggest that this procedure be performed daily, and it should always be done if the aneroid manometer was dropped or jostled. Unless legally prohibited, it is thus recommended that facilities keep at least one mercury manometer for such calibration checks. The setup of the calibration system is shown in *Figure 3.1* and simply consists of a Y tube with the bottom end attached to a hand bulb and the top ends attached to both manometers. Note that the standard here is the mercury manometer.

The first step is to verify that both manometers are reading zero when there is no pressure being applied to the hand bulb. The next step in the process involves gently pumping the hand bulb so that the pressure reads 200 mm Hg on the mercury manometer. At this point, the reading of the aneroid manometer is recorded. The pressure is then released in approximately 30 mm Hg increments (*i.e.*, 170, 140, 110, 80, 50), with simultaneous aneroid manometer recordings being made at each interval.

If the readings are identical between the two manometers, the aneroid unit is considered perfectly calibrated. If there is a difference between the two manometers and the difference is consistent, the aneroid unit can still be used with a correction factor (*e.g.*, if there was always a reading of 6 mm Hg more for the aneroid gauge, then readings made with this unit would need to have 6 mm Hg subtracted). If, however, the readings between the two manometers are variable and >4 mm Hg, then the aneroid unit should not be used until repaired.

It is also important to regularly check the rubber bladder, tubing, and bulb for leaks because these develop as rubber ages and cracks. The pressure control valve on the hand bulb can also wear out and require replacement. Because of these common issues with BP equipment, it is recommended that facilities have replacement supplies readily available.

Assessment Technique

For accurate resting BP readings, it is important that the client be made as comfortable as possible. As with many other physiological and psychological measures taken on people, there exists what is called the "white coat syndrome" in the measurement of BP. This white coat syndrome refers to an elevation of BP because of the effect of being in a doctor's office or in a clinical setting (*i.e.*, clinician wearing a white lab coat). The recommended standardized procedures for assessing resting BP are listed in *Box 3.2*.

When an individual is beginning to learn the skill of BP measurement, it is helpful to work with an experienced technician who can listen with the trainee by using a dual head (two sets of listening tubes/earpieces) or teaching stethoscope as shown in *Figure 3.2*. Some helpful technique tips are as follows:

- Ideally, the client cuff should be applied to bare skin. However, thin clothing on the arm where the stethoscope is placed should not interfere with the measurement except for the slightly lower intensity of the sound. If clothing is between the

---

BOX 3.2   Procedures for Assessment of Resting Blood Pressure

1. Patients should be seated quietly for at least 5 min in a chair with back support (rather than on an examination table) with their feet on the floor and their arms supported at heart level. Patients should refrain from smoking cigarettes or ingesting caffeine for at least 30 min preceding the measurement.
2. Measuring supine and standing values may be indicated under special circumstances.
3. Wrap cuff firmly around upper arm at heart level; align cuff with brachial artery.
4. The appropriate cuff size must be used to ensure accurate measurement. The bladder within the cuff should encircle at least 80% of the upper arm. Many adults require a large adult cuff.
5. Place stethoscope chest piece below the antecubital space over the brachial artery. Bell and diaphragm side of chest piece appear equally effective in assessing BP (9).
6. Quickly inflate cuff pressure to 20 mm Hg above first Korotkoff sound.
7. Slowly release pressure at rate equal to 2–5 mm Hg $\cdot$ s^{-1}.
8. SBP is the point at which the first of two or more Korotkoff sounds is heard (phase 1), and DBP is the point before the disappearance of Korotkoff sounds (phase 5).
9. At least two measurements should be made (minimum of 1 min apart) and the average should be taken.
10. BP should be measured in both arms during the first examination. Higher pressure should be used when there is consistent interarm difference.
11. Provide to patients, verbally and in writing, their specific BP numbers and BP goals.

BP, blood pressure; DBP, diastolic blood pressure; SBP, systolic blood pressure.
Modified from (21). For additional, more detailed recommendations, see (18).

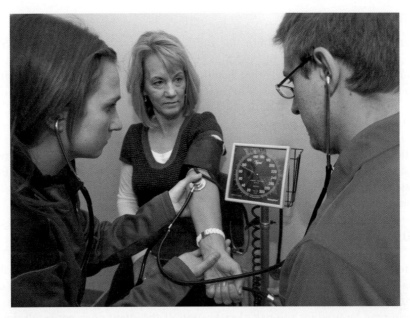

■ **FIGURE 3.2.** Use of a double-headed stethoscope used for training technicians learning to measure blood pressure. (Photograph by Ball State University.)

arm and the stethoscope and it is difficult to hear the Korotkoff sounds, then the procedure should be repeated with the arm bared. Note: as a general rule, avoid rolling up the client's sleeve if the clothing becomes too tight on the upper arm because this can influence the BP due to partial occlusion of the blood vessel.

- Locate the client's brachial artery (position with the palm up and arm rotated outward on the thumb side with the arm hyperextended). This artery, and thus pulse, is just medial to the biceps tendon. Mark the artery with an appropriate marker (watercolor) for the stethoscope bell placement, especially if the BP will be assessed again during exercise.
- Firmly place the bell of the stethoscope over the brachial artery. Avoid placing the bell of the stethoscope under the lip of the BP cuff.
- The stethoscope earpieces should be facing forward, toward the nose, in the same direction as the ear canal. (Note: If a stethoscope is being shared, the earpieces should be cleaned between users.)
- Position the manometer (either mercury or aneroid) so that the manometer is clearly visible and at eye level to avoid any parallax (distortion from looking up or down) error.
- After identifying the SBP, the pressure can be lowered ≈20 mm Hg rapidly and then slowed to the standard deflation rate of 2–5 mm Hg · s^{-1}. More rapid deflation leads to errors in the identification of DBP.
- Record both the fourth and fifth phase sounds if clearly heard. Always record only even numbers and round off upward to the nearest 2 mm Hg. Always continue to listen for any BP sounds for at least 10 mm Hg below the fifth phase.
- If needed, it is possible to increase the intensity, or loudness, of the brachial pulse sounds by either having the client raise the arm and rapidly make a tight fist and then relax the hand 5–10 times, or hold the arm overhead for 60 s. Immediately inflate the cuff after either of these procedures.

INTERPRETATION

As noted in *Table 2.1*, the criteria for the hypertension risk factor are an SBP of ≥140 mm Hg and/or a DBP of ≥90 mm Hg. Remember that high readings need to be confirmed by at least one other reading on a separate day. Also note that only physicians can make a diagnosis of hypertension. Fitness professionals should inform clients if their BP is elevated in the hypertensive range and recommend they follow up with their health care provider.

More detailed classifications of resting BP readings are found in *Table 3.1*. These classifications, which are from the "Seventh Report of the National High Blood Pressure Education Program" (4), also contain recommendations for patient follow-up. Fitness professionals should be familiar with at least the recommendations contained in the executive summary of this report.

BLOOD TESTS

To determine the presence of two of the coronary disease risk factors, hypercholesterolemia and prediabetes, a recent fasted blood test is required. Some clients who obtain regular physical examinations from their physicians may have had a recent test. If so, this value can be used for the risk classification. If the client does not recall the exact test values, a copy of the blood test report may need to be acquired from the health care provider.

Unfortunately, many American adults do not know their cholesterol and glucose values. Indeed, awareness in America regarding indicators and facts about diabetes and heart disease remains inadequate. The American Diabetes Association recently conducted a survey to test diabetes knowledge and concluded that "many Americans have very limited understanding of the basic facts about diabetes, as well as the

TABLE 3.1. Classification and Management of Blood Pressure for Adults[a]

BP Classification	SBP (mm Hg)	DBP (mm Hg)	Lifestyle Modification	Initial Drug Therapy	
				Without Compelling Indication	With Compelling Indications
Normal	<120	And <80	Encourage		
Prehypertension	120–139	Or 80–89	Yes	No antihypertensive drug indicated	Drug(s) for compelling indications[b]
Stage 1 hypertension	140–159	Or 90–99	Yes	Antihypertensive drug(s) indicated	Drug(s) for compelling indications[b] Other antihypertensive drugs, as needed
Stage 2 hypertension	≥160	Or ≥100	Yes	Antihypertensive drug(s) indicated Two-drug combination for most[c]	

[a]Treatment determined by highest BP category.

[b]Compelling indications include heart failure, postmyocardial infarction, high coronary heart disease risk, diabetes mellitus, chronic kidney disease, and recurrent stroke prevention. Treat patients with chronic kidney disease or diabetes mellitus to BP goal of <130/80 mm Hg.

[c]Initial combined therapy should be used cautiously in those at risk for orthostatic hypotension.

BP, blood pressure; DBP, diastolic blood pressure; SBP, systolic blood pressure.

Adapted from (21).

serious consequences for health that accompany the disease" (1). Awareness of cholesterol levels is lacking as well, and this is particularly true among specific sub-populations. For example, about one in five Latinos have high blood cholesterol yet only half of those with this condition know it (12). Among women, a recent survey conducted by the Society for Women's Health Research reported that although 79% knew how much they weighed in high school, only 32% knew their cholesterol level (21% for 18–44 yr olds and 43% for 55 yr and older) (23). The health risk assessment thus presents an opportunity to raise awareness of these risk factors and their implications on health.

The fitness professional has a couple of simple solutions if cholesterol and glucose values are unknown. One, a contract with a local laboratory that provides these blood-testing services can be obtained and then clients can be referred to this facility for testing. Another variation is to actually collect the blood sample from the client and then send the sample to the laboratory for analysis. The second option is to actually purchase the instrumentation for performing these tests. Many small, relatively economical systems are available commercially and offer the ability to perform cholesterol and glucose testing (and possibly other useful tests). Then both collection and testing of the sample can be performed on-site. Generally, such results are available for interpretation within minutes.

BLOOD SAMPLING METHODS

Phlebotomy is the practice of withdrawing blood from a blood vessel into a blood collection tube. Typically, this is done either by inserting a needle into a vein (larger volume sample) or by puncturing a finger (smaller volume sample). The venipuncture method is obviously more involved and thus requires a skilled phlebotomist to perform the task. There are professional phlebotomy training courses available because this skill is needed in all medical facilities and can involve advanced skills such as starting intravenous access lines; obtaining samples from arteries; and drawing samples from infants, children, and adults with characteristics that make the blood draw challenging. Fortunately, the sample needed for the cholesterol and glucose measures can be acquired by drawing a sample from an arm vein. There are modified courses that can provide training limited to this purpose. Some states have regulations that restrict the practice of phlebotomy to those with a defined level of training; thus, the state department of health should be contacted to determine if training and licensing regulations exist.

For facilities that purchase their own mini-sample systems, the blood sample can be obtained by a finger puncture as shown in *Figure 3.3*. This skill is much simpler and requires less training. In most cases, an automated device is placed on the finger and then triggered to puncture the skin. Indeed, all individuals with diabetes are trained to perform this technique because they need to regularly self-monitor their blood glucose levels. The sample may be collected into a small capillary tube, or the drop of blood that forms on the finger may be applied directly to a reagent pad depending on the instrumentation used.

STANDARD PRECAUTIONS

All health care and allied health care professionals should be trained to protect themselves against exposure to blood-borne pathogens. Indeed, the Occupational Safety and Health Administration (OSHA) of the Department of Labor has set national standards for these protections called Standard Precautions. A federal law (29 CFR

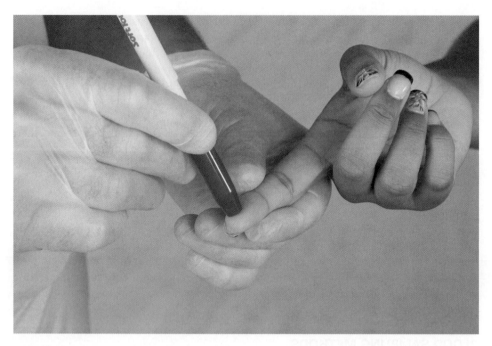

■ **FIGURE 3.3.** A device used to puncture the finger to obtain a blood sample. *Note:* Protective gloves would be worn by the technician.

1910.1030) was enacted in 1991 and provides the requirements for training and regular reviews of the procedures that should be followed to protect employees from the risks of exposure to blood-borne pathogens (25). Modifications to this law were further introduced in 2000 with The Needlestick Safety and Precaution Act (Pub L 106-430) (15). Certainly, all workers who will be involved in handling blood are required to have this training. However, it is reasonable for all fitness professionals who work with clients to assume they may be at risk of exposure to blood (*e.g.*, an accident that results in a cut of the skin) or possibly other bodily fluids (with the exception of sweat). Thus, it is prudent for all fitness professionals to obtain training in standard precautions and be familiar with the laws regarding blood-borne pathogens.

INTERPRETATION

Regardless of how the fitness professional obtains the blood test information, it is important to know how to interpret the results. The National Cholesterol Education Program has standardized the interpretation of results of cholesterol, including high-density lipoprotein (HDL), low-density lipoprotein (LDL), and triglycerides (10). *Table 3.2* provides these classifications. Refer back to *Chapter 2* for the criteria for the positive risk factor of hypercholesterolemia and the negative risk factor of high HDL. Likewise, the American Diabetes Association has set the standards that have become uniformly accepted in health care for interpretation of fasting blood glucose (2). The risk factor criteria (prediabetes) are values from 100 to 125 mg $\cdot$ dL^{-1}. Values <100 mg $\cdot$ dL^{-1} are considered normal, and values ≥126 mg $\cdot$ dL^{-1} are considered diagnostic for diabetes. Remember, as with resting BP measures, elevated values should be confirmed by at least one other test.

TABLE 3.2. ATP III Classification of LDL, Total, and HDL Cholesterol (mg · dL^{-1})

LDL Cholesterol	
<100[a]	Optimal
100–129	Near optimal/above optimal
130–159	Borderline high
160–189	High
≥190	Very high
Total Cholesterol	
<200	Desirable
200–239	Borderline high
≥240	High
HDL Cholesterol	
<40	Low
≥60	High
Triglycerides	
<150	Normal
150–199	Borderline high
200–499	High
≥500	Very high

[a]According to the American Heart Association/American College of Cardiology 2006 update (endorsed by the National Heart, Lung, and Blood Institute), it is reasonable to treat LDL cholesterol to <70 mg · dL^{-1} (<1.81 mmol · L^{-1}) in patients with coronary and other atherosclerotic vascular disease (22).

NOTE: To convert LDL, total cholesterol, and HDL from mg · dL^{-1} to mmol · L^{-1}, multiply by 0.0259. To convert triglycerides from mg · dL^{-1} to mmol · L^{-1}, multiply by 0.0113.

ATP III, Adult Treatment Panel III; HDL, high-density lipoprotein cholesterol; LDL, low-density lipoprotein cholesterol.

Adapted from (24).

OBESITY

Obesity was once thought to only affect coronary artery disease (CAD) through its impact on the other risk factors such as diabetes, hypertension, and hyperlipidemia. In other words, obesity was considered to be a primary factor leading to diabetes, hypertension, and hyperlipidemia, but only a secondary factor for CAD. This changed in 1998 when the American Heart Association, based on its review of the scientific literature, declared that obesity should be considered a major, independent risk factor for CAD (5).

Obesity is defined as an excessive amount of body fat. The assessment of body composition, which involves estimating body fat percentage, is the focus of *Chapter 4* of this manual. From a risk factor assessment perspective, obesity is determined from evaluating an individual's body weight compared to his or her height and also considering the girth of the abdominal region of the body. The term **overweight** is used as classification for body weights that are above what is considered the normal range for one's height yet below the criteria for obesity.

MEASUREMENT OF HEIGHT AND WEIGHT

Height is measured with an instrument called a stadiometer. A stadiometer consists of a vertical ruler, which is typically mounted to a wall, with a sliding horizontal

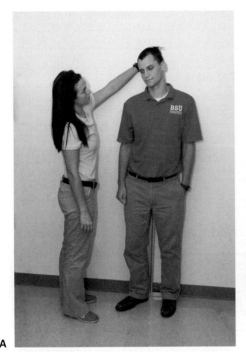
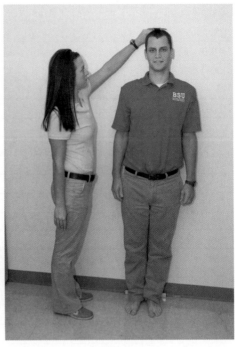

A   **B**

■ **FIGURE 3.4. A.** Incorrect technique used to measure height with a stadiometer; notice shoes are on, feet are not together, head is turned to the side, and the chin is tilted down. **B.** Correct technique. This is the standardized technique used to measure height with a stadiometer. (Photograph by Ball State University.)

platform. When mounted to a wall, calibration becomes unnecessary because the measurement scale is fixed in place. Portable units and vertical rods attached to weight scales are also available; however, if these are used, then the stadiometer scale readings should be checked with a vertical ruler placed on the platform prior to each measurement session. Although height is a simple and relatively routine measurement to perform, the following important standardization steps as highlighted in *Figure 3.4A* and *B* should be used:

- The client must remove shoes and hat (if worn).
- The client should stand erect with feet flat on the floor with heels touching each other.
- If using a wall-mounted stadiometer, the heels, midbody, and upper body parts should be touching the wall.
- The client should inhale normally and hold it while looking straight ahead (head in a neutral position relative to the chin).
- The horizontal headboard should be lowered to touch the top of the head (skull).

Weight can be measured with various types of scales with different mechanisms. One of the most popular types is the balance beam scale. Regardless of the type of scale used, the accuracy of the mechanism should be checked regularly. Most scales provide a method to calibrate the zero point. Checking the scale with no weight on it is an essential step prior to each measurement. If the scale is not reading 0 as shown in *Figure 3.5*, it should be adjusted to set the reading to 0. Some electronic scales also

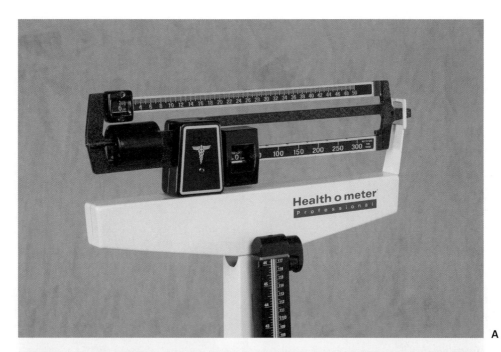

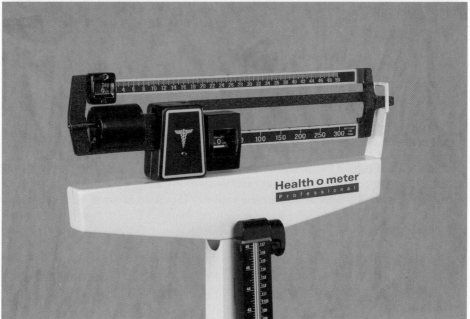

■ **FIGURE 3.5. A.** A correctly calibrated balance beam scale. **B.** A scale needing calibration of the zero point.

allow for a measurement of a standard amount of weight as a secondary check for accuracy. Ideally, this standard weight should be in the range of weights you expect for your clients; however, a smaller amount of weight is commonly used because it is more practical. Some electronic scales may have the ability to adjust the scale if the standardized weight reading is deviant from the scale reading, thereby calibrating the

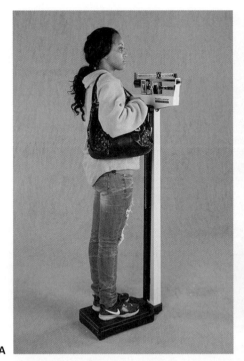
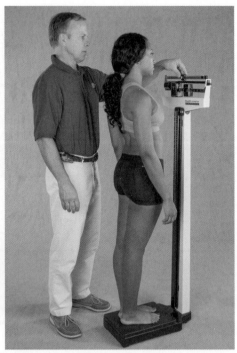

A

B

■ **FIGURE 3.6. A.** Incorrect technique used to measure weight; notice the shoes are on, the patient is fully clothed and wearing a coat. **B.** Correct standardized technique used to measure weight.

scale at this weight. However, most scales do not have this second adjustment setting and will require professional service to restore accuracy. A calibration check log sheet, recording the date and zero and standard weight readings, should be kept by the fitness professional. Fortunately, most high-quality weight scales maintain their calibration quite well. The fitness professional still needs to regularly perform calibration checks to confirm the accuracy of clients' body weight readings. Like height, measuring weight is simple and relatively routine. To obtain accurate measurements, the following important standardization steps as highlighted in *Figure 3.6A* and *B* should be used:

- Clients should wear minimal clothing. In fitness assessment programs, this is generally considered shorts and a T-shirt (no shoes). However, in other settings with "street clothes," the client should be instructed to remove any outer layers and shoes and also empty all pockets.
- The client should void the bladder prior (within 1 h) to the measurement.
- Ideally, weight should be measured in the morning prior to any meal or beverage consumption. However, because this is not always practical, the time of day should be similar for sequential measurement comparisons with no excess meal and beverage consumption prior to the measurement.

To track body weight over time, it is essential to follow the discussed standardizations. However, for screening programs, variations in the mentioned standards are acceptable with the understanding that the measured weight will be different from the standardized body weight.

Calculation of BMI

Body mass index (BMI), also called the Quetelet Index, is the weight-to-height ratio used to assess the obesity risk factor. This index compares an individual's weight (in kilograms) to his or her height (in meters squared). For example, an individual who weighs 150 lb and is 68 in tall would have a BMI calculated as follows:

Convert pounds to kilograms: 165 lb / 2.2046 lb/kg = 74.8 kg
Convert inches to centimeters: 68 in $\times$ 2.54 cm/in = 172.7 cm
Convert centimeters to meters: 172.7 cm / 100 cm/m = 1.727 m
Square the meter measure: 1.727 m $\times$ 1.727 m = 2.98 m^2
Calculate BMI: 74.8 kg / 2.98 m^2 = 25.1 kg $\cdot$ m^{-2}

Setting this formula up in a spreadsheet is a simple task and allows fitness professionals the ability to rapidly calculate BMI from height and weight measurements. Also, there are many Web sites such as the one hosted by the Obesity Education Initiative of the National Heart, Lung, and Blood Institute that provide online calculators of BMI (11).

MEASUREMENT OF WAIST CIRCUMFERENCE

The pattern of body weight distribution is recognized as an important predictor of health risks of obesity. Thus, the measurement of waist circumference is used as another indicator of obesity. This measurement identifies those with the abdominal type of obesity associated with greater health risk. The waist circumference is typically measured at the smallest circumference above the umbilicus and below the xiphoid process. This measurement should be performed using the following important standardization steps as highlighted in *Figure 3.7A* and *B*:

- The technician should stand on the right side of the client.
- The measurement should be made on bare skin.
- The measurement should be taken at the end of a normal exhalation by the client.
- The measuring tape should be parallel to the floor and should be pulled to lay flat on the skin without compressing the skin (some measurement tapes have a gauge to standardize the tension).
- Multiple measurements should be taken to determine the smallest circumference site. The mean of two measurements at this location (that do not differ by more than 1 cm) is used.

An alternative measurement site was proposed by the National Heart, Lung, and Blood Institute (13) and is shown in *Figure 3.8*. This site standardizes the location at just above the uppermost lateral border of the right iliac crest in line with the midaxillary line.

Some have advocated the additional measurement of the hip circumference to assess body fat distribution. The two circumference values are used to determine the waist-to-hip ratio (WHR). The hip circumference is measured as the largest circumference around the buttocks, above the gluteal fold (posterior extension), following the same standardization procedures used for waist measurement.

INTERPRETATION

The classifications for the obesity risk factor were provided in *Chapter 2*. Note that either (not necessarily both) an elevated BMI ($\geq$30 kg $\cdot$ m^{-2}) or increased waist

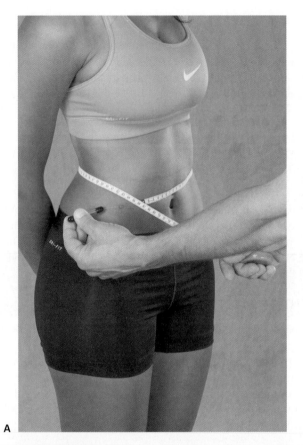

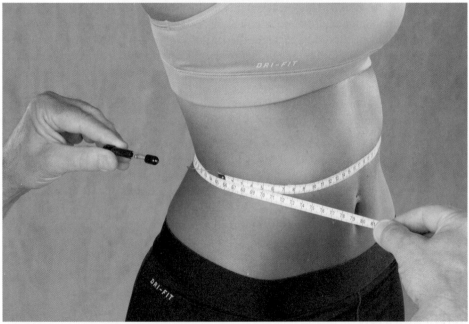

■ **FIGURE 3.7. A.** Incorrect technique used to measure waist circumference; notice the professional is standing in front of the client and the tape is not parallel to the floor. **B.** Correct standardized technique used to measure waist circumference.

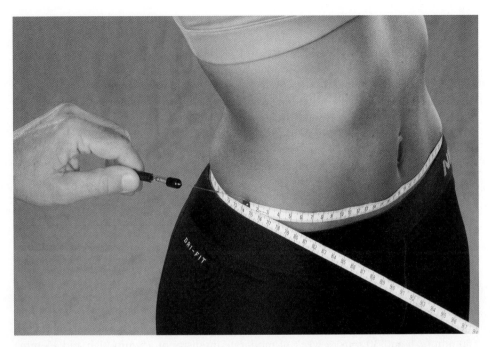

■ **FIGURE 3.8.** Measuring tape position for waist (abdominal) circumference using the alternative measurement site.

circumference (>88 cm for women or >102 cm for men) is used as the criterion for the obesity risk factor (14). Interestingly, there now appears to be some conflicting research regarding this BMI risk classification within patients diagnosed with heart failure. Recent studies have reported improved survival in this population when BMI is ≥ 30 kg $\cdot$ m^{-2}, a phenomenon known as the "obesity paradox" (3,16). The reasons for this paradox are unclear at present (1). Additional classifications of BMI status and disease risk can be obtained by using *Table 3.3*. Also, further detail and information on other classifications for the waist circumference and the WHR is provided within *Chapter 4* of *ACSM's GETP9*.

TABLE 3.3. Classification of Disease Risk Based on Body Mass Index (BMI) and Waist Circumference

		Disease Risk[a] Relative to Normal Weight and Waist Circumference	
	BMI (kg $\cdot$ m^{-2})	Men, ≤102 cm Women, ≤88 cm	Men, >102 cm Women, >88 cm
Underweight	<18.5	—	—
Normal	18.5–24.9	—	—
Overweight	25.0–29.9	Increased	High
Obesity, class			
I	30.0–34.9	High	Very high
II	35.0–39.9	Very high	Very high
III	≥40.0	Extremely high	Extremely high

It must be noted that the BMI scale is not a perfect marker for obesity. Some individuals may have a BMI of <30 kg $\cdot$ m^{-2} and could have excess body fat, and some individuals may have a BMI of ≥ 30 kg $\cdot$ m^{-2} and could have normal body fat levels. For the latter case, asking a few questions about adult body weight history and involvement in any activities related to heavy lifting (occupational or exercise) should help determine the potential for a misclassification. Clients who report significant weight gain in adulthood without any corresponding increase in heavy lifting activities have probably experienced weight gain comprised mostly of body fat, and the obesity classification is probably accurate. If significant doubt exists, the client could be referred for a body composition assessment.

PHYSICAL ACTIVITY

Physical activity represents one of the components of total daily energy expenditure, the other components being resting metabolic rate and the thermic effect of food. The voluntary nature of physical activity makes it the most variable component of total daily energy expenditure. Given the numerous health benefits of regular physical activity (26), public health guidelines have emerged regarding the recommended intensity and volume of physical activity necessary to promote health. Specifically, these guidelines advocate that inactivity should be avoided and that adults should obtain at least 150 min (2 h and 30 min) a week of moderate intensity or 75 min (1 h and 15 min) a week of vigorous intensity aerobic physical activity, or an equivalent combination of moderate and vigorous intensity aerobic activity (26). The guidelines further state that these physical activity targets can be obtained by accumulating bouts of activity throughout the day in smaller increments, such as 8- to 10-min durations. Given these recommendations, it is important to accurately assess the intensity, frequency, duration, and type of physical activity of an individual along with inactivity or sedentary time. This assessment becomes particularly critical when objectives involve refining the physical activity dose and health response relationship, investigating determinants to physical activity behavior, or evaluating intervention efforts to increase individual and population levels of physical activity.

From a risk assessment perspective, the highest interest lies in identifying those who are not meeting recommended amounts of physical activity (*i.e.*, inactive or irregularly active). Recall from *Table 2.1* that the criterion for defining the risk factor of sedentary lifestyle was *not participating in at least 30 min of moderate intensity, physical activity (40%–<60% $\dot{V}O_2R$) on at least 3 d of the week for at least 3 mo.* Generally, the assessment of physical activity can be broken down into either subjective assessment methods or objective assessment methods.

SUBJECTIVE ASSESSMENT

Subjective assessment methods include physical activity questionnaires, diaries, or logs. The level of detail can range from a four-item questionnaire attempting to distinguish overall global levels of activity (low vs. high levels) to a more detailed approach inquiring about different domains of activity (occupational, household, etc.) and the intensity, duration, frequency, and type of activity. There are many questionnaires that have been developed to assess physical activity.

The short version of the International Physical Activity Questionnaire (IPAQ), found in *Box 3.3*, is one that is relatively simple to use and can be completed by a client in about a minute (7). The instructions are straightforward, and the list of

BOX 3.3	International Physical Activity Questionnaire (7)

We are interested in finding out about the kinds of physical activities that people do as part of their everyday lives. The questions will ask you about the time you spent being physically active in the **last 7 days**. Please answer each question even if you do not consider yourself to be an active person. Please think about the activities you do at work, as part of your house and yard work, to get from place to place, and in your spare time for recreation, exercise or sport.

Think about all the **vigorous** activities that you did in the **last 7 days**.
Vigorous physical activities refer to activities that take hard physical effort and make you breathe much harder than normal.
Think *only* about those physical activities that you did for at least 10 minutes at a time.

1. During the **last 7 days**, on how many days did you do **vigorous** physical activities like heavy lifting, digging, aerobics, or fast bicycling?

    _____ **days per week** → How much time in total did you usually spend on one of these days doing vigorous physical activities?

    or   _____ **hours** _____ **minutes**

    none

Think about all the **moderate** activities that you did in the **last 7 days**. **Moderate** activities refer to activities that take moderate physical effort and make you breathe somewhat harder than normal.
Think only about those physical activities that you did for at least 10 minutes at a time.

2. During the **last 7 days**, on how many days did you do **moderate** physical activities like carrying light loads, bicycling at a regular pace, or doubles tennis? Do not include walking.

    _____ **days per week** → How much time in total did you usually spend on one of these days doing moderate physical activities?

    or   _____ **hours** _____ **minutes**

    none

Think about the time you spent **walking** in the **last 7 days**.
This includes at work and at home, walking to travel from place to place, and any other walking that you might do solely for recreation, sport, exercise, or leisure.

3. During the **last 7 days**, on how many days did you **walk** for at least 10 minutes at a time?

    _____ **days per week** → How much time in total did you usually spend on one of these days doing walking on one of those days?

    or   _____ **hours** _____ **minutes**

    none

The last question is about the time you spent **sitting** on weekdays during the **last 7 days**.

BOX 3.3	International Physical Activity Questionnaire (7) (*Continued*)

Include time spent at work, at home, while doing course work and during leisure time. This may include time spent sitting at a desk, visiting friends, reading, or sitting or lying down to watch television.

4. During the **last 7 days**, how much time did you spend **sitting** on a **weekday**?

_____ **hours** _____ **minutes**

This is the end of the questionnaire, thank you.

examples of physical activities can be modified to fit the background of the client completing the questionnaire. The IPAQ uses a variable called metabolic equivalent (MET) $\cdot$ min $\cdot$ wk^{-1} for determining classifications. MET $\cdot$ min $\cdot$ wk^{-1} is calculated by multiplying the MET level for the type of activity by the number of minutes that activity was performed per day by the number of days per week the activity was performed. Walking is scored as 3.3 METs, moderate intensity activities are scored as 4 METs, and vigorous intensity activities are scored as 8 METs. For example, a person who reported performing moderate intensity activity for 30 min per day for 5 d of the week would have obtained 600 MET $\cdot$ min $\cdot$ wk^{-1} (4 METs $\times$ 30 min $\cdot$ d^{-1} $\times$ 5 d $\cdot$ wk^{-1}). Physical activity level classifications from the IPAQ assessment are shown in *Table 3.4*.

OBJECTIVE ASSESSMENT

Objective assessment methods include assessment tools such as motion sensors (*i.e.*, pedometers/step counters and accelerometers as shown in *Fig. 3.9*), heart rate monitoring, and combination-type approaches (*i.e.*, accelerometer plus heart rate monitoring plus temperature). These types of monitors are typically worn on the body. For instance, pedometers/step counters and accelerometers can be worn at the level of the hip or ankle, heart rate monitors typically involve wearing a heart rate chest band and a watch-type receiver, and some combination monitors can be worn on the arm or at

TABLE 3.4. Physical Activity Level Classifications from an International Physical Activity Questionnaire (IPAQ) Assessment (8)	
Category 1 (Low)	Not active enough to meet criteria for categories 2 or 3
Category 2 (Moderate)	$\geq$3 d of vigorous activity of $\geq$20 min $\cdot$ d^{-1} OR $\geq$5 d of moderate-intensity activity or walking of $\geq$30 min $\cdot$ d^{-1} OR $\geq$5 d of any combination of walking or moderate- or vigorous-intensity activities achieving a minimum of 600 MET $\cdot$ min $\cdot$ wk^{-1}
Category 3 (High)	Vigorous-intensity activity $\geq$3 d $\cdot$ wk^{-1}, achieving at least 1,500 MET $\cdot$ min $\cdot$ wk^{-1} OR 7 d of any combination of walking or moderate- or vigorous-intensity activities achieving a minimum of 3,000 MET $\cdot$ min $\cdot$ wk^{-1}

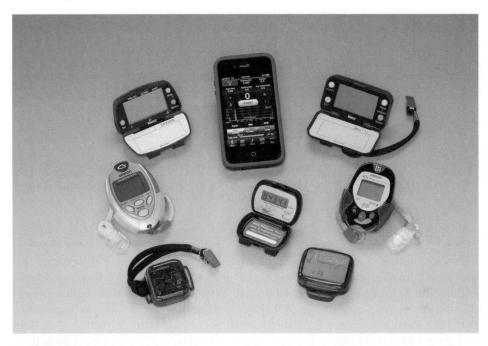

■ **FIGURE 3.9.** Many different models of pedometers and accelerometers are available to objectively measure physical activity.

the hip. Manufacturers of these devices typically specify the chosen location to wear such devices. Objective monitors are usually small, lightweight, and unobtrusive.

The advantages and disadvantages of subjective and objective methods of assessing physical activity are outlined in *Table 3.5*. In choosing a physical activity assessment tool, be aware of the individual advantages and disadvantages of the method, and match the tool chosen to the needs of the assessment. In most risk classification situations, it is advantageous to acquire immediate assessment of the client's physical activity behavior. In this instance, a paper questionnaire may be the tool of choice. However,

TABLE 3.5. Comparison of Objective and Subjective Physical Activity Assessment Tools

	Objective Assessment	Subjective Assessment
Advantages	Concurrent measure of activity — as one moves, it measures and records it Able to continuously record data for multiple days and weeks at a time Has an internal time clock, so activity can be time-stamped to a specific time of day	Inexpensive Can be tailored to specific populations Can be administered to a large population
Disadvantages	Expensive Unable to determine type of activity May not capture nonambulatory activity (cycling, weightlifting)	Error from self-report (memory) and self-perception (intensity) Poor in assessing typical activities of daily living (*i.e.*, lifestyle activities)

TABLE 3.6. Classification of Physical Activity Behavior (26)	
Inactive	No activity beyond baseline activities of daily living.
Low activity	Activity beyond baseline but fewer than 150 min (2 h and 30 min) of moderate-intensity physical activity a week or the equivalent amount (75 min, or 1 h and 15 min) of vigorous-intensity physical activity
Medium activity	150 min to 300 (5 h) min of moderate-intensity physical activity a week (or 75–150 min of vigorous-intensity physical activity a week). In scientific terms, this range is approximately equivalent to 500–1,000 metabolic equivalent (MET) minutes a week.
High activity	More than the equivalent of 300 min of moderate-intensity physical activity a week

with some advanced planning, objective monitors can be employed. Many facilities now offer assessments with accelerometers to obtain data on total inactivity time and time spent in light, moderate, and vigorous activities. Accelerometer reports can also provide information on bouts of moderate-to-vigorous intensity that last at least 10 min in duration. To capture the volatile nature of a person's physical activity with an objective assessment tool, a minimum period of observation is needed. It is recommended that these monitors be worn from the time the person wakes up in the morning until they go to bed at night. Valid observation days should have at least 12 hr of wear time. Assessing physical activity for a minimum of 3 weekdays and at least 1 weekend day is recommended, although longer monitoring periods (1–2 wk) are optimal.

INTERPRETATION

There can be numerous outcomes after assessing an individual's physical activity level, and this often depends on the assessment method chosen. For instance, some activity questionnaires may output calories expended; others will output an index range of 1–4, 1 being low active and 4 being the most active. Accelerometers may output the number of minutes a person spends being inactive and in light, moderate, or vigorous intensity activity on a daily basis, whereas a pedometer/step counter will yield the total number of steps taken on a particular day. Many of these output units are not interchangeable, or they become less valid in conversion. For instance, an attempt to convert steps accumulated per day into calories expended per day will result in the loss of some measurement accuracy. The validity of the method chosen and the selected output variable should always be considered when measuring physical activity levels.

Interpreting an individual's physical activity level can establish a profile of behavior and classify the person as either engaging in enough activity to be health enhancing or engaging in so little activity as to warrant a classification of sedentary or inactive. Seasonal variation is also evident in physical activity behavior and needs to be considered when assessing and comparing physical activity patterns. *Table 3.6* presents a classification system of physical activity behavior.

OTHER DISEASES AND CONDITIONS

There are other health-related issues that can easily be included in a screening, particularly if the program is a comprehensive health-based program. Although these issues related to the HRPF assessment are less common, some fitness professionals will offer these services.

PULMONARY DISEASE

There are many types of pulmonary (lung) diseases, some of which can manifest early in life (*e.g.*, asthma). Among the list of indications for pulmonary function testing (*Table 3.7A*) are

- to evaluate all smokers older than the age of 45 yr,
- to assess health status before beginning strenuous physical activity programs, and
- to evaluate symptoms (*e.g.*, dyspnea [shortness of breath], chronic cough, wheezing, or excessive mucus production).

Because some HRPF assessments require vigorous-to-maximal exertion, identifying those with abnormal pulmonary function would be valuable. Testing of pulmonary function can involve many different tests with specialized equipment that need to be administered by professionals with training in these procedures. However, there is a basic test that can be administered in screening programs that requires little equipment and can be conducted at a reasonable cost. The test requires the client to perform a maximal inhalation, followed by maximally exhaling as rapidly as possible. The total amount of air expelled in this procedure is called the forced vital capacity (FVC). The equipment used to measure the FVC will also measure the amount of air expelled in the first second of the procedure. This volume of air is called the forced expiratory volume in one second ($FEV_{1.0}$). It is common to use the ratio of these two variables, $FEV_{1.0}$/FVC, as the primary screening measure, with any value below 70% considered below normal limits. The interpretation can become more detailed as noted in *Table 3.7B*. Those interested in more detailed interpretations should review the section on pulmonary function testing in *Chapter 3* of the *ACSM's GETP9*.

OSTEOPOROSIS

Osteoporosis is a disease that is characterized by low bone mass and structural deterioration of bone tissue, which is often accompanied by bone fractures. Although often thought of as a condition seen primarily in elderly women, the National Osteoporosis Foundation (NOF) estimates that osteoporosis is a major health threat for 55% of Americans older than age 50 yr. Public awareness of the causes and consequences of the disease is critical as NOF asserts that "osteoporosis is often considered a pediatric disease with geriatric consequences – approximately 85–90 percent of adult bone mass is acquired by age 18 in girls and 20 in boys" (14).

The definitive test for diagnosing osteoporosis is a bone scan with a dual-energy X-ray absorptiometer (DXA), which is typically only available in clinical and research facilities. However, the fitness professional can administer a survey to help identify those who may be at greater risk. A version of a short, easy-to-administer and -interpret survey from the NOF is shown in *Box 3.4*.

SUMMARY

Many fitness professionals can provide a valuable service by offering measurements of several different factors related to risk classification assessment. These additional measurements do require specialized training and some instrumentation. Minimally, the fitness professional should know resources in the community where these services can be obtained and needs to be knowledgeable about the interpretation of the results from these risk factor assessments.

TABLE 3.7. Indications for Spirometry

A. Indications for Spirometry

Diagnosis

To evaluate symptoms, signs, or abnormal laboratory tests

To measure the effect of disease on pulmonary function

To screen individuals at risk of having pulmonary disease

To assess preoperative risk

To assess prognosis

To assess health status before beginning strenuous physical activity programs

Monitoring

To assess therapeutic intervention

To describe the course of diseases that affect lung function

To monitor individuals exposed to injurious agents

To monitor for adverse reactions to drugs with known pulmonary toxicity

Disability/Impairment Evaluations

To assess patients as part of a rehabilitation program

To assess risks as part of an insurance evaluation

To assess individuals for legal reasons

Public Health

Epidemiologic surveys

Derivation of reference equations

Clinical research

B. The Global Initiative for Chronic Obstructive Lung Disease Spirometric Classification of COPD Severity Based on Postbronchodilator $FEV_{1.0}$

Stage I	Mild	$FEV_{1.0}/FVC < 0.70$
		$FEV_{1.0} \geq 80\%$ of predicted
Stage II	Moderate	$FEV_{1.0}/FVC < 0.70$
		$50\% \leq FEV_{1.0} < 80\%$ predicted
Stage III	Severe	$FEV_{1.0}/FVC < 0.70$
		$30\% \leq FEV_{1.0} < 50\%$ predicted
Stage IV	Very severe	$FEV_{1.0}/FVC < 0.70$
		$FEV_{1.0} < 30\%$ predicted or $FEV_{1.0} < 50\%$ predicted plus chronic respiratory failure

C. The American Thoracic Society and European Respiratory Society Classification of Severity of Any Spirometric Abnormality Based on $FEV_{1.0}$

Degree of Severity	$FEV_{1.0}$ % Predicted
Mild	Less than the LLN but ≥ 70
Moderate	60–69
Moderately severe	50–59
Severe	35–49
Very severe	< 35

| BOX 3.4 | Are You at Risk of Osteoporosis? |

OSTEOPOROSIS: CAN IT HAPPEN TO YOU?

Osteoporosis is a major public health threat for 44 million Americans. Ten million individuals already have osteoporosis and 34 million more have low bone mass placing them at increased risk for developing osteoporosis and the fractures it causes. Estimates suggest that about half of all women older than 50, and up to one in four men, will break a bone because of osteoporosis. Known as "the silent thief," osteoporosis progresses without symptoms or pain until bones start to break, generally in the hip, spine, or wrist. Learn more about this bone-thinning disease that causes serious fractures.

Complete the questionnaire to determine your risk for developing osteoporosis.

Yes No

❑ ❑ Is your calcium intake low? (*e.g.*, Do you eat less than three servings of dairy products or calcium-fortified foods per day without taking a calcium supplement?)

❑ ❑ Is your vitamin D intake low? (*e.g.*, Do you eat few, if any, sources of vitamin D like milk and fish, without taking a vitamin D supplement?)

❑ ❑ Do you perform less than 2.5 hours of weight-bearing or endurance exercise per week? (*e.g.*, brisk walking, taking aerobics classes, playing tennis, dancing and hiking)

❑ ❑ Do you perform muscle-strengthening or resistance exercise less than twice a week? (*e.g.*, lifting weights or gardening)

❑ ❑ Do you smoke cigarettes?

Yes No

❑ ❑ Do you consume more than two alcoholic drinks per day?

❑ ❑ Are you age 50 or older?

❑ ❑ Are you a postmenopausal woman?

❑ ❑ If yes, did you go through menopause before age 45?

❑ ❑ Did either of your parents have osteoporosis?

❑ ❑ Are you small and thin?

❑ ❑ Have you broken a bone after the age of 50?

❑ ❑ Have you lost an inch or more in height?

❑ ❑ Is your spine curving forward?

❑ ❑ Have you ever taken medicines* that can lead to osteoporosis?

❑ ❑ Have you ever been diagnosed with a medical condition* that can lead to osteoporosis?

*For a list of medicines and medical conditions that can lead to osteoporosis, please visit www.nof.org.

The more times you answer "yes," the greater your risk for developing osteoporosis. See your health care provider and contact the National Osteoporosis Foundation (NOF) for more information. Osteoporosis is a complex disease and not all of its causes are known. However, when certain risk factors are present, your likelihood of developing osteoporosis is increased. Therefore, it is important for you to determine your risk of developing osteoporosis and take action to prevent it now.

Osteoporosis is preventable if bone loss is detected early. If the questions suggest that you are at risk for developing osteoporosis, see your health care provider. Your health care provider may recommend that you have a bone mass measurement test. This test will safely and accurately measure your bone density and reliably predict your risk of future fracture.

If you already have osteoporosis, you can live actively and comfortably by seeking proper medical care and making some adjustments to your lifestyle. Your health care provider may prescribe a diet rich in calcium and vitamin D, a regular program of weight-bearing exercise, and medical treatment.

| BOX 3.4 | Are You at Risk of Osteoporosis? (*Continued*) |

NOF is the nation's leading authority for patients and health care providers seeking up-to-date, medically sound information and educational materials on the causes, prevention, detection, and treatment of osteoporosis. Please contact NOF at www. nof.org for more information or to find out how you can join in the fight against this devastating disease.

LABORATORY ACTIVITIES

RESTING BLOOD PRESSURE ASSESSMENT

Data Collection
- Perform a calibration check of the aneroid manometer you will use for the laboratory. Record the results of this calibration check and provide an interpretation.
- Measure eight students' resting BP and allow eight students to measure your resting BP following the procedures in *Box 3.2*. Record the values that were measured on you below (do not let the technician see the previous measurement values).

Technician	1	2	3	4	5	6	7	8
SBP								
DBP								

Written Report
1. Graph the data and comment on the variability in the measurements. Provide a critique of any deviations from recommended techniques you observed from watching the technicians. Using the mean values for SBP and DBP, provide an interpretation of your resting BP.
2. Provide responses for the following:
   - Describe the white coat syndrome.
   - Explain how the principle of the auscultatory method is used for BP assessment.
   - Which of the Korotkoff sounds is used for SBP? What phase of the Korotkoff sounds is TRUE DBP?

BODY MASS INDEX ASSESSMENT

Data Collection
- Perform any necessary calibration check of the equipment and report your findings.
- Measure eight students' height, weight, and waist circumference and allow eight students to make these measures on you following the procedures in this manual. Record the values that were measured on you below (do not let the technician see the previous measurement values). Calculate the BMI (show your work on these calculations).

Technician	1	2	3	4	5	6	7	8
Height								
Weight								
BMI								
Waist								

Written Report

1. Graph the data and comment on the variability in the measurements. Provide a critique of any deviations from recommended techniques you observed from watching the technicians.
2. Using the mean values for height, weight, and waist circumference, provide an interpretation of your BMI and disease risk.

INTERNATIONAL PHYSICAL ACTIVITY QUESTIONNAIRE ASSESSMENT

Data Collection

- Complete a short-form IPAQ (*Box* 3.3).
- Ask two friends or relatives (one of each gender) who work full time to complete a short-form IPAQ.

Written Report

1. Perform the calculations of MET $\cdot$ min $\cdot$ wk^{-1} on each of these three physical activity assessments.
2. Provide interpretations of each of the three subjects' IPAQ physical activity classifications and explain the criteria you used to choose the classification category.

CASE STUDY

Jerome stopped by a booth that was a part of a health fair at the local mall. Jerome, who is 29 yr old, had never had his cholesterol measured. He had a fingerstick blood sample taken, which was analyzed for total cholesterol and HDL cholesterol. The results reported that his total cholesterol was 287 mg $\cdot$ dL^{-1} and his HDL was 43 mg $\cdot$ dL^{-1}, and it was recommended that he have the test repeated again on another day. Jerome knew that the ABC Fitness Center offered a service of performing lipid profiles, so he arranged to have a fasted blood test. The results from this test were total cholesterol, 265 mg $\cdot$ dL^{-1}; HDL, 38 mg $\cdot$ dL^{-1}; triglycerides, 185 mg $\cdot$ dL^{-1}; LDL, 190 mg $\cdot$ dL^{-1}; and glucose, 106 mg $\cdot$ dL^{-1}. Provide an interpretation of these tests and explain what recommendation you would make to Jerome.

REFERENCES

1. American Diabetes Association. As America earns failing grade, American Diabetes Association launches movement to stop diabetes. *American Diabetes Association Survey Finds* [Internet]. 2009 [cited 2011 Jul 15]. Available from: http://www.diabetes.org/for-media/2009/america-earns-failing-adm-sd-2009.html
2. American Diabetes Association. Standards of medical care in diabetes—2011. *Diabetes Care*. 2011;34:S11–61.
3. Arena R, Lavie CJ. The obesity paradox and outcome in heart failure: is excess bodyweight truly protective? *Future Cardiol*. 2010;6(1):1–6.

4. Chobanian AV, Bakis GL, Black HR, et al. The seventh report of the Joint National Committee on Prevention, Detection, Evaluation, and Treatment of High Blood Pressure. *JAMA*. 2003;289:2560–72.

5. Eckel RH, Krauss RM. American Heart Association call to action: obesity as a major risk factor for coronary heart disease. *Circulation*. 1998;86:340–44.

6. Executive summary of the clinical guidelines on the identification, evaluation, and treatment of overweight and obesity in adults. *Arch Intern Med*. 1998;158(17):1855–67.

7. International Physical Activity Questionnaire. Self-administered, short-form [Internet]. 2001 [cited 2011 Jul 15]. Available from: https://sites.google.com/site/theipaq/questionnaires

8. International Physical Activity Scoring Protocol [Internet]. Revised 2005 [cited 2011 Jul 20]. Available from: https://sites.google.com/site/theipaq/scoring-protocol

9. Kantola I, Vesalainen R, Kangassalo K, Kariluoto A. Bell or diaphragm in the measurement of blood pressure? *J Hypertens*. 2005;23(3):499–503.

10. National Cholesterol Education Program. Executive summary of the Third Report of the National Cholesterol Education Program (NCEP) Expert Panel on Detection, Evaluation, and Treatment of High Blood Cholesterol in Adults (Adult Treatment Panel III). *JAMA*. 2001;285:2486–97.

11. National Heart, Lung, and Blood Institute, U.S. Department of Health and Human Services. Aim for a healthy weight; BMI Calculator [Internet]. [cited 2011 Jul 15]. Available from: http://www.nhlbisupport.com/bmi

12. National Heart, Lung, and Blood Institute, U.S. Department of Health and Human Services. Do you know your cholesterol levels: Healthy hearts, healthy homes. NIH publication 08-6353 [Internet]. 2008 [cited 2011 Jul 15]. Available from: http://www.nhlbi.nih.gov/health/public/heart/other/latino/chol/cholesterol.pdf

13. National Institutes of Health, National Heart, Lung, and Blood Institute. *Clinical Guidelines on the Identification, Evaluation, and Treatment of Overweight and Obesity in Adults*. Bethesda (MD): National Heart, Lung, and Blood Institute; 1998. NIH publication 98-4083.

14. National Osteoporosis Foundation. News Release: National Osteoporosis Foundation releases new survey results during National Osteoporosis Awareness and Prevention Month [Internet]. 2011 [cited 2011 Jul 15]. Available from: http://www.nof.org/news/nofnews/2011-0501-NOFNews

15. Needlestick Safety and Precautions Act of 2000, Pub. L. No. 106–430, 114 Stat. 1901. *National Institute of Health* [Internet]. 2000 [cited 2011 Jul 15]. Available from: http://history.nih.gov/research/downloads/PL106–430.pdf

16. Oreopoulos A, Padwal R, Kalantar-Zadech K, Fonarow GC, Norris CM, McAlister FA. Body mass index and mortality in heart failure: a meta-analysis. *Am Heart J*. 2008;156(1):13–22.

17. Pellegrino R, Viegi G, Brusasco V, et al. Interpretative strategies for lung function tests. *Eur Respir J*. 2005; 26(5):948–68.

18. Pickering TG, Hall JE, Appel LJ, et al. Recommendations for blood pressure measurement in humans and experimental animals: Part 1: blood pressure measurement in humans: a statement for professionals from the Subcommittee of Professional and Public Education of the American Heart Association Council on High Blood Pressure Research. *Hypertension*. 2005;45(1):142–61.

19. Pickering TG, Miller NH, Ogedegbe G, Krakoff LR, Artinina NT, Goff D. Call to action on the use and reimbursement for home blood pressure monitoring. A joint statement from the American Heart Association, American Society of Hypertension, and Preventative Cardiovascular Nurses Association. *Hypertension*. 2008;52:10–29.

20. Rabe KF, Hurd S, Anzueto A, et al. Global strategy for the diagnosis, management, and prevention of chronic obstructive pulmonary disease: GOLD executive summary. *Am J Respir Crit Care Med*. 2007;176(6):532–55.

21. *The Seventh Report of the Joint National Committee on Prevention, Detection, Evaluation, and Treatment of High Blood Pressure (JNC7)* [Internet]. Bethesda (MD): National High Blood Pressure Education Program; 2004 [cited 2012 Jan 7]. 104 p. Available from: http://www.nhlbi.nih.gov/guidelines/hypertension

22. Smith SC Jr, Allen J, Blair SN, et al. AHA/ACC Guidelines. AHA/ACC guidelines for secondary prevention for patients with coronary and atherosclerotic vascular disease: 2006 update. *Circulation*. 2006;113:(19)2363–72.

23. Society For Women's Health. Older American women better informed about cholesterol than younger women but gaps remain in knowledge and screening [Internet]. 2007 [cited 2011 Jul 15]. Available from: http://www.womenshealthresearch.org/site/News2?page=NewsArticle&id=6993&news_iv_ctrl=-1

24. *Third Report of the National Cholesterol Education Program (NCEP) Expert Panel on Detection, Evaluation, and Treatment of High Blood Cholesterol in Adults (Adult Treatment Panel III)* [Internet]. Bethesda (MD): National Cholesterol Education Program; 2004 [cited Mar 19]. 284 p. Available from: http://www.nhlbi.nih.gov/guidelines/cholesterol/index.htm

25. United States Department of Labor, Occupational Safety & Health Administration. Bloodborne pathogens regulations (Standards 29 CFR: 1910.1030) [Internet]. 1991 [cited 2011 Jul 15]. Available from: http://www.osha.gov/pls/oshaweb/owasrch.search_form?p_doc_type=STANDARDS&p_toc_level=0&p_keyvalue=

26. U.S. Department of Health and Human Services Physical Activity Guidelines for Americans. *2008 Physical Activity Guidelines for Americans* [Internet]. Washington (DC): U.S. Department of Health and Human Services; 2008 [cited 2011 Jul 15]. Available from: http://www.health.gov/paguidelines/

27. U.S. Environmental Protection Agency. Mercury. Information for Health care providers [Internet]. 2010 [cited 2011 Jul 11]. Available from: http://www.epa.gov/hg/healthcare.htm#facilities

Body Composition

WHY MEASURE BODY COMPOSITION?

In the most general sense, body composition is the study of the components of the body and their relative proportions. There is clinical value to knowing the amount of these varied body components. For example, the total amount (mass) and density of bone tissue is a critical measure to assess in the diagnosis and prognosis of osteoporosis. From a health-related physical fitness (HRPF) assessment point of view, body composition is defined as the relative proportions of fat and fat-free tissue in the body, typically expressed as a total body fat percentage. Historically, the focus of HRPF body composition assessments has been to obtain estimates of body fat percentage. Although percentage of fat is still the primary outcome variable, more attention is beginning to be paid to determining the amount, or percentage, of muscle mass.

HEALTH IMPLICATIONS

In *Chapters* 2 and 3, the risks of obesity, as measured by body mass index (BMI) and waist circumference, were discussed. As a result of the high prevalence of obesity, many fitness professionals emphasize body composition assessment to their clients. However, the opposite end of the spectrum, low levels of body fat, also merits recognition. This is particularly relevant for girls and young women who are at greater risk for developing eating disorders and all athletes who are involved in sports where weight impacts performance. Unless clinically indicated, the assessment of body composition is typically not recommended for those with or at risk for developing an eating disorder.

It is also important to recognize changes in health-related components of body composition that accompany aging. Sarcopenia is defined as the age-related loss of muscle mass, with accompanying decreases in strength. Although precise measurement of the total amount of muscle mass is not obtained in the HRPF body composition assessment, it is a major component of the fat-free tissue that is estimated, and as such should be reported. Indeed, it is important to recognize that it is the muscle mass that is most directly related to both muscular and cardiorespiratory fitness.

FUNCTIONAL IMPLICATIONS

Both obesity and sarcopenia result in some degree of functional impairment for individuals. Often, younger individuals are not as concerned about the accompanying health risks of conditions such as obesity and coronary heart disease because these do not seem relevant to their daily lives. Yet evidence shows that obesity rates in children and youth have tripled between 1980 and 2008 (6). Explaining and discussing the functional limitations of obesity may be a key in promoting an understanding of the negative effects of obesity. Such a discussion may encourage involvement in a fitness program.

Sarcopenia is increasingly being targeted as a major predictor of disability, resulting in nursing home institutionalization for older adults. Many adults perform only limited amounts of activities requiring high levels of muscular power, and most have neglected any forms of resistance exercise training. Thus, assessment of estimates of amount of muscle mass should be considered in assessments because these results may be of value to older adults and actually provide motivation to incorporate muscular fitness training into their exercise programs.

WHAT IS THE GOLD STANDARD TEST?

The simple, straightforward answer to the preceding question is that no method exists to accurately quantify the total amount of body fat in a living individual. Some clinical measures, as will be discussed in the next section, can provide accurate determinations of the amount of body fat in particular segments of the body. However, more investigations are needed prior to applying these expensive technologies in the determination of total body fat percentage.

Historically, the method of underwater (hydrostatic) weighing has been considered a gold standard for body fat percentage assessments. This method, used to determine body density (Db), has typically been employed as the standard against which other methods are compared. An overview of underwater weighing is provided later in this chapter.

CLINICAL MEASURES

Fitness professionals will have limited ability to obtain clinical measures of body composition for their clients. However, some clients may obtain these measures as part of their medical care and may bring the results to the fitness professional for advice.

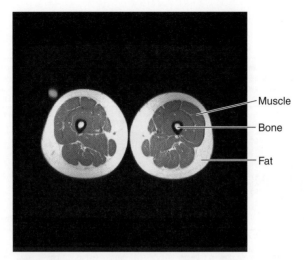

■ **FIGURE 4.1.** A magnetic resonance imaging scan of the thighs of a 30-yr-old woman. Source: Ball State University — Dr. Todd Trappe.

MAGNETIC RESONANCE IMAGING AND COMPUTED TOMOGRAPHY

Magnetic resonance imaging (MRI) and computed tomography (CT) scans are typically used as diagnostic procedures for various different diseases. These devices take a cross-sectional picture (think of this as one thin slice) of a region of the body. Recently, scientists have used these technologies to assess the change in amount of fat, bone, and muscle tissue related to different interventions, including exercise. *Figure 4.1* shows an MRI scan of a segment of the thighs of a 30-yr-old woman. *Figure 4.2* shows a CT scan of a segment of the abdomen in an older man. Note the layer of subcutaneous fat on both of these scans. In these experimental research studies, the scientists will take a scan at the same location before and after the intervention and then accurately measure the change in tissue at this segment of the body.

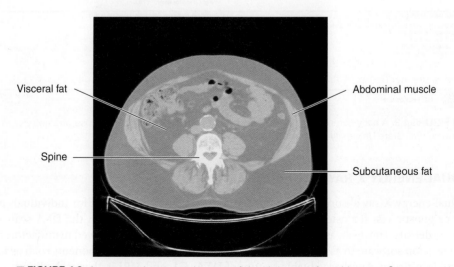

■ **FIGURE 4.2.** A computed tomography scan of the abdomen of an older man. Source: Ball State University — Dr. Todd Trappe.

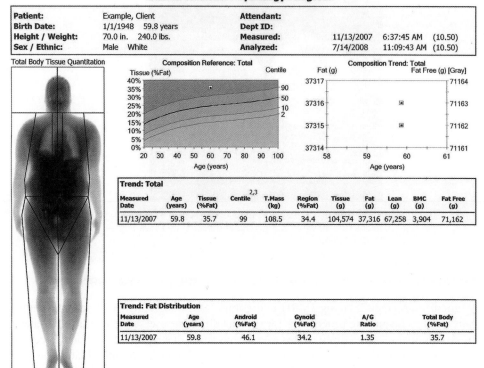

■ FIGURE 4.3. A body composition report from a total body dual-energy X-ray absorptiometry scan. Source: Ball State University — Clinical Exercise Physiology Program.

DUAL-ENERGY X-RAY ABSORPTIOMETRY

Dual-energy X-ray absorptiometry (DXA) measurements are ordered for individuals as a diagnostic test for osteoporosis. The main outcome measure from the DXA scan is bone density. However, as X-ray technology has improved, it has allowed manufacturers to develop software to assess the relative amounts of other body components such as fat and lean tissue. Another valuable feature of DXA, CT, and MRI is that each allows the evaluation of regional body fat proportions. *Figure 4.3* shows an example of one total body DXA scan and the body composition report.

Ball State University
Human Performance Laboratory
Clinical Exercise Physiology Program

Patient:	Example, Client		Attendant:			
Birth Date:	1/1/1948 59.8 years		Dept ID:			
Height / Weight:	70.0 in. 240.0 lbs.		Measured:	11/13/2007	6:37:45 AM	(10.50)
Sex / Ethnic:	Male White		Analyzed:	7/14/2008	11:09:43 AM	(10.50)

BODY COMPOSITION

Region	Tissue (%Fat)	Region (%Fat)	Tissue (g)	Fat (g)	Lean (g)	BMC (g)	Total Mass (kg)
Left Arm	26.0	24.8	5,264	1,371	3,893	260	-
Left Leg	31.8	30.4	15,430	4,904	10,526	714	-
Left Trunk	41.4	40.4	28,830	11,923	16,908	684	-
Left Total	35.6	34.4	52,680	18,780	33,900	1,981	-
Right Arm	26.0	24.9	5,314	1,383	3,931	252	-
Right Leg	31.8	30.5	15,511	4,935	10,575	688	-
Right Trunk	41.4	40.4	28,294	11,706	16,588	708	-
Right Total	35.7	34.4	51,894	18,536	33,358	1,923	-
Arms	26.0	24.8	10,578	2,754	7,824	512	-
Legs	31.8	30.4	30,941	9,839	21,102	1,402	-
Trunk	41.4	40.4	57,125	23,628	33,496	1,393	-
Android	46.1	45.7	10,249	4,720	5,529	84	-
Gynoid	34.2	33.3	15,827	5,414	10,413	416	-
Total	35.7	34.4	104,574	37,316	67,258	3,904	108.5

FAT MASS RATIOS

Trunk/ Total	Legs/ Total	(Arms+Legs)/ Trunk
0.63	0.26	0.53

3 -Matched for Age, Weight (males 25-100 kg), Ethnic

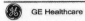 GE Healthcare

Lunar Prodigy
DF+10199

■ **FIGURE 4.3.** (*Continued*)

TESTS OF BODY VOLUME

The measurement of volume is used to determine density with the formula:

$$Density = mass/volume$$

Different types of body tissues have different density values. From an HRPF body composition assessment perspective, the known difference in the density of fat versus fat-free tissues is used to derive estimates of body fat percentage. Mass, or body weight, can be accurately determined following the procedures outlined in *Chapter 3*. Two widely used HRPF body composition assessment methods — underwater weighing and plethysmography — allow for a determination of body volume. These methods are discussed in detail in the next section.

Once volume has been derived, Db is then used to estimate body fat percentage. The following two commonly used generalized equations are those developed by Siri (9) and Brozek et al. (2).

Siri equation:

$$\text{Body fat (\%)} = (495/\text{Db}) - 450$$

Brozek equation:

$$\text{Body fat (\%)} = (457/\text{Db}) - 414.2$$

However, as more research has been performed on individuals with different characteristics, population-specific equations have been developed and are shown in *Table 4.1*. These equations were developed around the knowledge that body mass can be differentiated on two components: fat mass (FM) and fat-free mass (FFM).

UNDERWATER (HYDROSTATIC) WEIGHING

The underwater weighing method of determining body volume is based on Archimedes' principle, which states that a body immersed in a fluid is buoyed up by a force equal to the weight of the displaced fluid. This method measures body volume via water displacement. To determine body volume using the underwater weighing method requires measurements of body weight before entering the water and the loss of body weight when submerged underwater. The underwater weight is influenced by two amounts of air trapped in the body; residual lung volume and gas in the gastrointestinal (GI) system. This trapped air contributes to buoyancy and thus needs to be factored into the calculation of underwater weight. Ideally, residual volume should be measured; however, it is often predicted, and a constant value of 100 mL is used for GI gas. The following common formulas are used to estimate residual volume based on gender, height (cm), and age:

Men: Residual volume (L) = $[0.019 \cdot \text{height (cm)}] + [0.0155 \cdot \text{age (years)}] - 2.24$ (1)

Women: Residual volume (L) = $[0.032 \cdot \text{height (cm)}] + [0.009 \cdot \text{age (years)}] - 3.90$ (7)

Also, because the density of the water varies with temperature, the temperature of the water needs to be measured. The density of water at a specific temperature can be determined using a Web site provided by SiMetric.co.uk (10).

Typically, a freestanding tank of water is used for the underwater weighing procedure. Within the tank is a chair for seating the client, which is attached to a scale for weight measurement as depicted in *Figure 4.4*. The assessment procedures for underwater weighing are provided in *Box 4.1*. Owing to the effort requirement to maximally exhale while being submerged underwater, the results of this test are dependent on the client's effort and success in performing the technique correctly. The formula for calculating body volume from this procedure is:

$$\text{Body volume} = (\{[\text{Body weight (g)} - \text{Underwater weight (g)}]/ \text{Water density (g/cm}^3)\} - [\text{Residual volume (mL)} + 100 \text{ mL}])$$

Finally, body weight is divided by body volume to derive Db.

TABLE 4.1. Population-Specific Formulas for Conversion of Body Density to Percent Body Fat

	Population	Age	Gender	%BF	FFBd[a] (g · cm⁻³)
ETHNICITY	African American	9–17	Women	$(5.24 / Db) - 4.82$	1.088
		19–45	Men	$(4.86 / Db) - 4.39$	1.106
		24–79	Women	$(4.86 / Db) - 4.39$	1.106
	American Indian	18–62	Men	$(4.97 / Db) - 4.52$	1.099
		18–60	Women	$(4.81 / Db) - 4.34$	1.108
	Asian Japanese Native	18–48	Men	$(4.97 / Db) - 4.52$	1.099
			Women	$(4.76 / Db) - 4.28$	1.111
		61–78	Men	$(4.87 / Db) - 4.41$	1.105
			Women	$(4.95 / Db) - 4.50$	1.100
	Singaporean (Chinese, Indian, Malay)		Men	$(4.94 / Db) - 4.48$	1.102
			Women	$(4.84 / Db) - 4.37$	1.107
	Caucasian	8–12	Men	$(5.27 / Db) - 4.85$	1.086
			Women	$(5.27 / Db) - 4.85$	1.086
		13–17	Men	$(5.12 / Db) - 4.69$	1.092
			Women	$(5.19 / Db) - 4.76$	1.090
		18–59	Men	$(4.95 / Db) - 4.50$	1.100
			Women	$(4.96 / Db) - 4.51$	1.101
		60–90	Men	$(4.97 / Db) - 4.52$	1.099
			Women	$(5.02 / Db) - 4.57$	1.098
	Hispanic		Men	NA	NA
		20–40	Women	$(4.87 / Db) - 4.41$	1.105
ATHLETES	Resistance trained	24 ± 4	Men	$(5.21 / Db) - 4.78$	1.089
		35 ± 6	Women	$(4.97 / Db) - 4.52$	1.099
	Endurance trained	21 ± 2	Men	$(5.03 / Db) - 4.59$	1.097
		21 ± 4	Women	$(4.95 / Db) - 4.50$	1.100
	All sports	18–22	Men	$(5.12 / Db) - 4.68$	1.093
		18–22	Women	$(4.97 / Db) - 4.52$	1.099
CLINICAL POPULATIONS[b]	Anorexia nervosa	15–44	Women	$(4.96 / Db) - 4.51$	1.101
	Cirrhosis				
	Childs A			$(5.33 / Db) - 4.91$	1.084
	Childs B			$(5.48 / Db) - 5.08$	1.078
	Childs C			$(5.69 / Db) - 5.32$	1.070
	Obesity	17–62	Women	$(4.95 / Db) - 4.50$	1.100
	Spinal cord injury (paraplegic/quadriplegic)	18–73	Men	$(4.67 / Db) - 4.18$	1.116
		18–73	Women	$(4.70 / Db) - 4.22$	1.114

[a]FFBd, fat-free body density based on average values reported in selected research articles.

[b]There are insufficient multicomponent model data to estimate the average FFBd of the following clinical populations: coronary artery disease, heart/lung transplants, chronic obstructive pulmonary disease, cystic fibrosis, diabetes mellitus, thyroid disease, HIV/AIDS, cancer, kidney failure (dialysis), multiple sclerosis, and muscular dystrophy.

%BF, percentage of body fat; Db, body density; NA, no data available for this population subgroup.

Adapted with permission from (4).

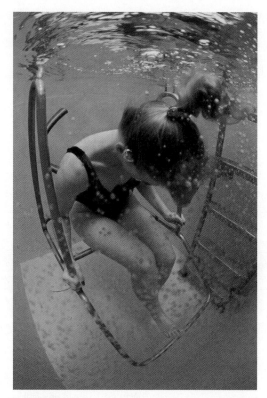

■ **FIGURE 4.4.** The underwater weighing procedure.

PLETHYSMOGRAPHY

As with hydrostatic weighing, plethysmography is also based on the concept of displacement; but in this procedure, the matter being displaced is air. A body plethysmograph can determine changes in volume (V) with measures of pressure (P) according to Boyle's law (P1V1 = P2V2, if temperature is constant). There is one leading manufacturer selling a whole body plethysmograph (the BOD POD) to provide measures of body volume by assessing air displacement. This plethysmograph has two chambers. Measurements of pressure and volume are first made with the front chamber empty, then with a standard cylinder of known volume to calibrate the system, and then finally with a person in the front chamber. The second, back chamber, remains closed at all times and simply serves as a reference chamber. The procedure requires the client to follow similar pretest standardizations as for underwater weighing (see *Box 4.1*). Additionally, the client must wear only tight-fitting clothing made of nylon (typically a swimsuit or cycling shorts and a jog bra) and a swim cap to control for temperature variations caused by hair on the head as shown in *Figure 4.5*. The client only needs to remain still while the instrument makes the measures of body volume, thus making this procedure less demanding and time consuming than underwater weighing. The outcome measure of body volume is then used to calculate Db.

ANTHROPOMETRY

Anthropometry is the measurement of the human body, which includes measures of circumferences or girths as well as skinfolds. Anthropometric measurements are made at various specific sites on the body.

| BOX 4.1 | Procedures for Underwater Weighing |

PRETEST STANDARDIZATIONS
1. Clients should be in a normally hydrated state and should not have eaten for at least 3 h.
2. Immediately prior to the assessment, clients should empty the bladder and attempt to empty the bowels.
3. Clients should remove any makeup, body oils, and jewelry prior to entering the water.
4. Clients should wear a tight-fitting swimsuit to eliminate air trapping.
5. Explain to clients that they should begin exhaling as they gently submerge themselves under the water and to continue exhaling as much as possible. At that point, they need to remain underwater as long as possible and remain as still as possible to obtain a stable underwater weight reading. This procedure will need to be repeated multiple times (typically 5–10) as there is generally a learning effect for this procedure.

ASSESSMENT PROCEDURES
1. Obtain a body weight measurement on clients before they enter the water.
2. Measure the temperature of the water.
3. Have clients enter the water and sit on the suspended chair.
4. Have clients submerge themselves underwater, following the instructions provided. Note: Some clients may require that the chair be weighted if while performing the procedure, a part of their body breaks the surface of the water (because of buoyancy).
5. Repeat step 4 until at least three consecutive underwater weight readings do not increase.

SKINFOLD MEASUREMENTS

Skinfold measurements can be used to estimate body fat percentage based on the assumption that the amount of subcutaneous fat is proportional to the total amount of body fat. At first glance, pinching a fold of skin and applying a set of calipers to measure the distance appears to be a simple skill. However, consistently obtaining accurate skinfold measurements requires a good quality skinfold caliper, specific training, and a significant amount of practice.

The skinfold caliper should deliver a specific amount of force ($12g \cdot mm^{-2}$), and good-quality calipers come with this assurance from the manufacturer. *Figure 4.6* provides examples of the range in quality of skinfold calipers available. One source of variability in skinfold measurement occurs from using a caliper that does not deliver the recommended amount of force. Ideally, this level of force should be checked periodically; however, because most facilities lack the necessary instrumentation to do this, it is seldom done. The caliper distance measurement should also be checked using a simple standardized calibrations block as shown in *Figure 4.7*.

The skinfold procedure requires that the technician grasp the skin with the thumb and index finger approximately 3 in (7.5 cm) apart and firmly pull the skin, with the underlying subcutaneous fat, away from the limb or torso. The fold will contain two

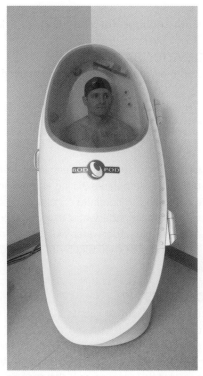

■ **FIGURE 4.5.** A client having his body
fat percentage estimated using whole
body plethysmography.

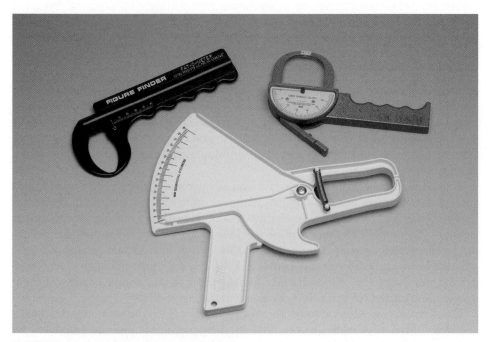

■ **FIGURE 4.6.** Range in quality of skinfold calipers.

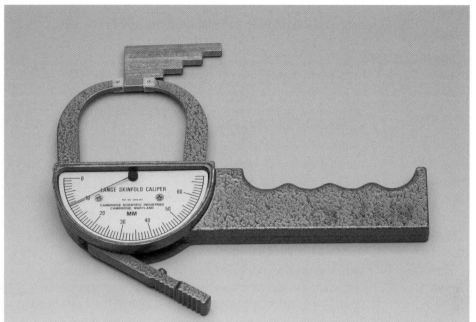

A

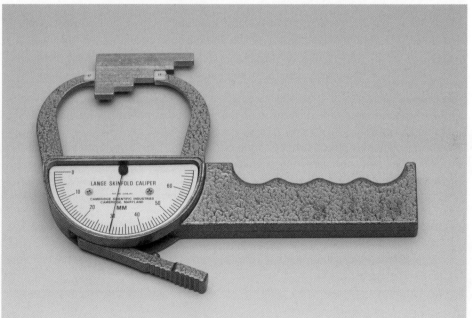

B

■ **FIGURE 4.7.** The method to check the distance calibration of a pair of skinfold calipers.

layers of skin with only fat in between. If there is any doubt about the fold containing some muscle tissue, the client should be instructed to contract the muscle at that site to allow the technician to feel whether any muscle exists in the fold. The arms of the caliper are opened and applied to the skinfold by gradually releasing the pressure on the caliper arms. Note that the measurement scale should be facing up for viewing, which for most calipers requires a right-handed grip. *Box 4.2* provides descriptions of

BOX 4.2	Standardized Description of Skinfold Sites and Procedures

SKINFOLD SITE

Abdominal	Vertical fold; 2 cm to the right side of the umbilicus
Triceps	Vertical fold; on the posterior midline of the upper arm, halfway between the acromion and olecranon processes, with the arm held freely to the side of the body
Biceps	Vertical fold; on the anterior aspect of the arm over the belly of the biceps muscle, 1 cm above the level used to mark the triceps site
Chest/Pectoral	Diagonal fold; one-half the distance between the anterior axillary line and the nipple (men), or one-third of the distance between the anterior axillary line and the nipple (women)
Medial calf	Vertical fold; at the maximum circumference of the calf on the midline of its medial border
Midaxillary	Vertical fold; on the midaxillary line at the level of the xiphoid process of the sternum. An alternate method is a horizontal fold taken at the level of the xiphoid/sternal border in the midaxillary line
Subscapular	Diagonal fold (at a 45-degree angle); 1–2 cm below the inferior angle of the scapula
Suprailiac	Diagonal fold; in line with the natural angle of the iliac crest taken in the anterior axillary line immediately superior to the iliac crest
Thigh	Vertical fold; on the anterior midline of the thigh, midway between the proximal border of the patella and the inguinal crease (hip)

Procedures

- All measurements should be made on the right side of the body with the subject standing upright
- Caliper should be placed directly on the skin surface, 1 cm away from the thumb and finger, perpendicular to the skinfold, and halfway between the crest and the base of the fold
- Pinch should be maintained while reading the caliper
- Wait 1–2 s (not longer) before reading caliper
- Take duplicate measures at each site and retest if duplicate measurements are not within 1–2 mm
- Rotate through measurement sites or allow time for skin to regain normal texture and thickness

the standardized skinfold sites along with procedural recommendations as shown in *Figure 4.8A–G*. Careful attention to the anatomic landmarks and the actual measurement of distances is important for obtaining accurate and reliable measures. Once the location is identified, it should be marked on the skin with a water-solvent ink pen. Variation in the location of the skinfold site and the application of the calipers create the largest sources of error in skinfold measures. *Figure 4.9A and B* illustrate examples of correct and incorrect procedures for skinfold assessments.

Because the proportion of subcutaneous to total fat is known to vary between genders, between ethnic groups, and with age, different prediction equations have

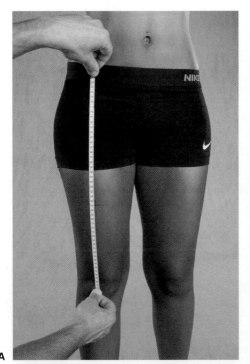
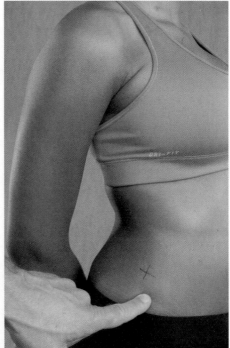
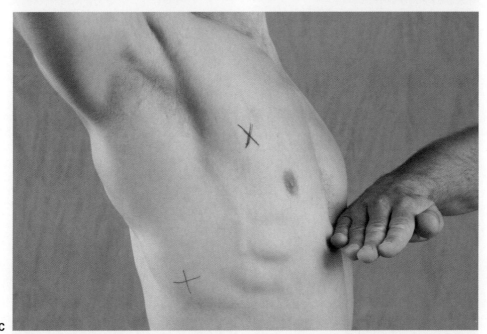

■ **FIGURE 4.8. A.** The thigh skinfold site. **B.** The suprailiac skinfold site. **C.** The midaxillary skinfold site. (*Continued*)

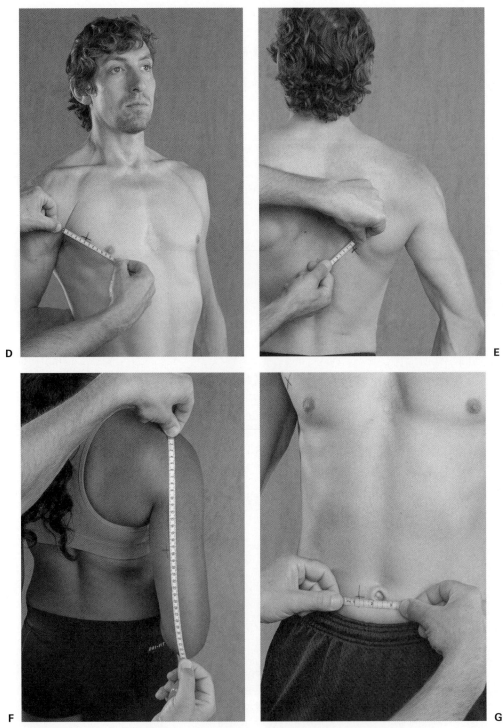

■ FIGURE 4.8. (*Continued*) **D.** The chest skinfold site. **E.** The subscapular skinfold site. **F.** The triceps skinfold site. **G.** The abdomen skinfold site.

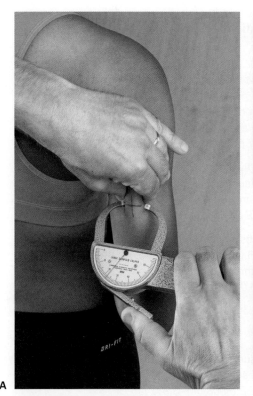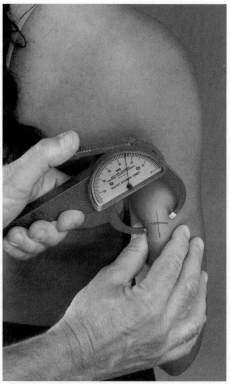

A B

■ **FIGURE 4.9. A.** Example of correct procedures for skinfold assessments. **B.** Example of incorrect procedures for skinfold assessments.

been developed to estimate body fat percentage. There are also generalized equations that can be used for most clients as well as specialized population-specific equations that can be used if working with a homogeneous group of people (*e.g.*, female collegiate volleyball players). The most commonly used method for estimating Db via skinfold measurement employs the generalized equations provided in *Box 4.3*. For both men and women, there are three options: one that uses seven and two that use three different skinfold sites (5,8). Theoretically, the more skinfold sites measured, the better the prediction of body fat. However, for most clients, there are minimal differences between the three- and seven-site methods, so the three-site methods are typically used.

CIRCUMFERENCES MEASUREMENTS

Circumference measurements have the advantages of being easily, inexpensively, and quickly administered. The only equipment requirement is an inexpensive measurement tape. Circumferences, also known as girths, are best used to measure changes in size of a body part. Perhaps the most important application is the use of circumferences to determine body fat distribution as was covered in *Chapter 3*. Circumferences can also be used to measure muscle girth size and therefore quantify changes in muscle with specific training (*e.g.*, resistance weight training) or to help monitor sarcopenia. Training and/or age-related muscle change measurements are most commonly measured in the limbs. For this purpose, measurement of the arm, forearm, midthigh, and calf are recommended.

BOX 4.3	Generalized Skinfold Equations

MEN

- **Seven-Site Formula** (chest, midaxillary, triceps, subscapular, abdomen, suprailiac, thigh)
  Body density = 1.112 − 0.00043499 (sum of seven skinfolds)
  + 0.00000055 (sum of seven skinfolds)^2
  − 0.00028826 (age) *[SEE 0.008 or ~3.5% fat]*

- **Three-Site Formula** (chest, abdomen, thigh)
  Body density = 1.10938 − 0.0008267 (sum of three skinfolds)
  + 0.0000016 (sum of three skinfolds)^2
  − 0.0002574 (age) *[SEE 0.008 or ~3.4% fat]*

- **Three-Site Formula** (chest, triceps, subscapular)
  Body density = 1.1125025 − 0.0013125 (sum of three skinfolds)
  + 0.0000055 (sum of three skinfolds)^2
  − 0.000244 (age) *[SEE 0.008 or ~3.6% fat]*

WOMEN

- **Seven-Site Formula** (chest, midaxillary, triceps, subscapular, abdomen, suprailiac, thigh)
  Body density = 1.097 − 0.00046971 (sum of seven skinfolds)
  + 0.00000056 (sum of seven skinfolds)^2
  − 0.00012828 (age) *[SEE 0.008 or ~3.8% fat]*

- **Three-Site Formula** (triceps, suprailiac, thigh)
  Body density = 1.099421 − 0.0009929 (sum of three skinfolds)
  + 0.0000023 (sum of three skinfolds)^2
  − 0.0001392 (age) *[SEE 0.009 or ~3.9% fat]*

- **Three-Site Formula** (triceps, suprailiac, abdominal)
  Body density = 1.089733 − 0.0009245 (sum of three skinfolds)
  + 0.0000025 (sum of three skinfolds)^2
  − 0.0000979 (age) *[SEE 0.009 or ~3.9% fat]*

SEE, standard error of estimate.
Adapted from (5,8).

There are some equations that use either circumferences or a combination of circumference and skinfold measurement to estimate body fat percentage (see *ACSM's GETP9 Chapter 4*); however, this approach is not commonly used. *Box 4.4* provides descriptions of the standardized circumference sites along with procedural recommendations.

BIOELECTRICAL IMPEDANCE ANALYSIS

One other method for estimating body fat percentage that has gained popularity in commercial fitness programs is the bioelectrical impedance analysis (BIA). The bioelectrical impedance analyzer introduces a small electrical current into the body and measures the resistance to that current as it passes through the body. Current will flow more readily through water in the body, which contains electrolytes. Fat contains only

BOX 4.4 Standardized Description of Circumference Sites and Procedures

Abdomen:
With the subject standing upright and relaxed, a horizontal measure taken at the height of the iliac crest, usually at the level of the umbilicus.

Arm:
With the subject standing erect and arms hanging freely at the sides with hands facing the thigh, a horizontal measure midway between the acromion and olecranon processes.

Buttocks/Hips:
With the subject standing erect and feet together, a horizontal measure is taken at the maximal circumference of buttocks. This measure is used for the hip measure in a waist/hip measure.

Calf:
With the subject standing erect (feet apart ~20 cm), a horizontal measure taken at the level of the maximum circumference between the knee and the ankle, perpendicular to the long axis.

Forearm:
With the subject standing, arms hanging downward but slightly away from the trunk and palms facing anteriorly, a measure is taken perpendicular to the long axis at the maximal circumference.

Hips/Thigh:
With the subject standing, legs slightly apart (~10 cm), a horizontal measure is taken at the maximal circumference of the hip/proximal thigh, just below the gluteal fold.

Mid-Thigh
With the subject standing and one foot on a bench so the knee is flexed at 90 degrees, a measure is taken midway between the inguinal crease and the proximal border of the patella, perpendicular to the long axis.

Waist:
With the subject standing, arms at the sides, feet together, and abdomen relaxed, a horizontal measure is taken at the narrowest part of the torso (above the umbilicus and below the xiphoid process). The National Obesity Task Force (NOTF) suggests obtaining a horizontal measure directly above the iliac crest as a method to enhance standardization. Unfortunately, current formulae are not predicated on the NOTF suggested site.

Procedures
- All measurements should be made with a flexible yet inelastic tape measure.
- The tape should be placed on the skin surface without compressing the subcutaneous adipose tissue.
- If a Gulick spring-loaded handle is used, the handle should be extended to the same marking with each trial.
- Take duplicate measures at each site and retest if duplicate measurements are not within 5 mm.
- Rotate through measurement sites or allow time for skin to regain normal texture.

Modified from (3).

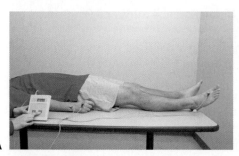
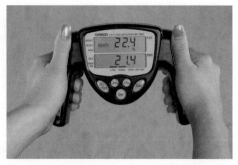

A   **B**

■ **FIGURE 4.10. A.** A bioelectrical impedance analysis (BIA) device that uses electrodes on the hand and foot. **B.** A handheld BIA device. (Photograph by Ball State University.)

small amounts of water, so current will not flow easily (*i.e.*, impeded) through areas containing fat. Conversely, lean tissue, which contains large amounts of water, and thus electrolytes, will be a good electrical conductor.

Because the BIA measure is dependent on total body water and is based on assumptions about water content of fat and lean tissues, anything that changes a person's hydration status will affect the prediction of body fat percentage. Patients who are prescribed a medication that has a diuretic property should avoid this test because the results will probably not be valid. To control for factors that affect hydration status, the following pretest conditions should be used prior to a BIA measurement:

- No alcohol consumption for the previous 48 h before the test
- No products with diuretic properties (*e.g.*, caffeine, chocolate) for the previous 24 h before the test
- No exercise for the previous 12 h before the test
- No eating or drinking for the previous 4 h before the test
- Bladder should be voided completely within 30 min of the test

The procedures for BIA measurement are specific to the actual BIA device that is being used as shown in *Figure 4.10A* and *B*. Calibration of most devices is limited to an internal system check. Some devices require placing electrodes on the hand and foot to collect the information. Others require a person to hold handles or stand on a platform to gather the information. There are no specific procedural requirements for the clients. Prior to the measurement, demographic data including age, gender, height, and weight are entered. Ideally, the client should have height and weight measured according to the procedures outlined in *Chapter 3*. Some of the BIA devices may also allow input of some category of physical activity status as well as ethnic/racial group. Similar to the skinfold method, BIA estimates of body fat percentage can be made from either generalized or population-specific equations, and some BIA devices allow the user to select an equation. Generally, most devices do not report the actual impedance values, so the raw data are unavailable for use in other equations.

INTERPRETATION

Normative standards for body fat percentage have not been developed in part because of the differences in measures between the various methods and variable standard errors of estimate (SEEs) for these methods. The American College of Sports Medicine (ACSM) uses the reference values established by the Cooper Institute, shown in

%		20–29	30–39	40–49	50–59	60–69	70–79
		Age (year)					
99	Very lean[a]	4.2	7.3	9.5	11.0	11.9	13.6
95		6.4	10.3	12.9	14.8	16.2	15.5
90	Excellent	7.9	12.4	15.0	17.0	18.1	17.5
85		9.1	13.7	16.4	18.3	19.2	19.0
80		10.5	14.9	17.5	19.4	20.2	20.1
75	Good	11.5	15.9	18.5	20.2	21.0	21.0
70		12.6	16.8	19.3	21.0	21.7	21.6
65		13.8	17.7	20.1	21.7	22.4	22.3
60		14.8	18.4	20.8	22.3	23.0	22.9
55	Fair	15.8	19.2	21.4	23.0	23.6	23.7
50		16.6	20.0	22.1	23.6	24.2	24.1
45		17.5	20.7	22.8	24.2	24.9	24.7
40		18.6	21.6	23.5	24.9	25.6	25.3
35	Poor	19.7	22.4	24.2	25.6	26.4	25.8
30		20.7	23.2	24.9	26.3	27.0	26.5
25		22.0	24.1	25.7	27.1	27.9	27.1
20		23.3	25.1	26.6	28.1	28.8	28.4
15	Very poor	24.9	26.4	27.8	29.2	29.8	29.4
10		26.6	27.8	29.2	30.6	31.2	30.7
5		29.2	30.2	31.3	32.7	33.3	32.9
1		33.4	34.4	35.2	36.4	36.8	37.2
n =		1,844	10,099	15,073	9,255	2,851	522

TABLE 4.2. Fitness Categories for Body Composition (% Body Fat) for Men by Age

Total *n* = 39,644

[a]Very lean, no less than 3% body fat is recommended for men.

Adapted with permission from *Physical Fitness Assessments and Norms for Adults and Law Enforcement.* The Cooper Institute, Dallas, Texas. 2009. For more information: www.cooperinstitute.org

Tables 4.2 and 4.3, for interpretation. It is important to recognize that these values are devised from only the population that was tested at the Cooper Institute. The values are expressed as percentiles for each 10-yr age group by gender. One concern with this approach is observed by comparing the 50th percentile for 20–29 yr olds (men 16.6% and women 21%) to that of 50–59 yr olds (men 22.7% and women 28.8%). Note the 6.1% and 7.8% increases for what is considered average between these age groups. There are known physiological changes in the composition of the body with age. For example, it is well accepted that bone mass and density will decline with age, particularly in postmenopausal women. However, many of the changes observed in different age groups in adult populations regarding body fat percentage may actually be attributed to changes in lifestyle (physical activity and diet) rather than to the physiological changes of aging. Thus the 50th percentile, although representing an average for a given population, does not necessarily represent a desirable value from a health and fitness standpoint. The *ACSM's GETP9* reports a criterion-based (as satisfactory

TABLE 4.3. Fitness Categories for Body Composition (% Body Fat) for Women by Age

%		20–29	30–39	40–49	50–59	60–69	70–79
				Age (year)			
99	Very lean[a]	11.4	11.2	12.1	13.9	13.9	11.7
95		14.0	13.9	15.2	16.9	17.7	16.4
90		15.1	15.5	16.8	19.1	20.2	18.3
85	Excellent	16.1	16.5	18.3	20.8	22.0	21.2
80		16.8	17.5	19.5	22.3	23.3	22.5
75		17.6	18.3	20.6	23.6	24.6	23.7
70	Good	18.4	19.2	21.7	24.8	25.7	24.8
65		19.0	20.1	22.7	25.8	26.7	25.7
60		19.8	21.0	23.7	26.7	27.5	26.6
55		20.6	22.0	24.6	27.6	28.3	27.6
50	Fair	21.5	22.8	25.5	28.4	29.2	28.2
45		22.2	23.7	26.4	29.3	30.1	28.9
40		23.4	24.8	27.5	30.1	30.8	30.5
35		24.2	25.8	28.4	30.8	31.5	31.0
30	Poor	25.5	26.9	29.5	31.8	32.6	31.9
25		26.7	28.1	30.7	32.9	33.3	32.9
20		28.2	29.6	31.9	33.9	34.4	34.0
15		30.5	31.5	33.4	35.0	35.6	35.3
10	Very poor	33.5	33.6	35.1	36.1	36.6	36.4
5		36.6	36.2	37.1	37.6	38.2	38.1
1		38.6	39.0	39.1	39.8	40.3	40.2
n =		1,250	4,130	5,902	4,118	1,450	295

Total n = 17,145

[a]Very lean, no less than 10%–13% body fat is recommended for women.

Adapted with permission from *Physical Fitness Assessments and Norms for Adults and Law Enforcement.* The Cooper Institute, Dallas, Texas. 2009. For more information: www.cooperinstitute.org

for health) range of 10%–22% body fat for men and 20%–32% body fat for women. However, there is limited data to support any true criterion-based approach for interpreting body fat results.

As discussed in *Chapter 1*, whenever an assessment is based on estimation, the interpretation should include an expression of the SEE. *Table 4.4* provides the SEE values for hydrostatic weighing, plethysmography, skinfolds, and BIA.

TABLE 4.4. Standard Error of Estimate for Different Body Fat Assessment Methods

Method for Estimating Body Fat Percentage	Standard Error of Estimate
Air displacement (BOD POD)	±2.2% to ±3.7%
Bioelectrical impedance analysis	±3.5% to ±5%
Dual-energy X-ray absorptiometry	±1.8%
Skinfold measurements	±3.5%
Underwater weighing	±2.5%

Adapted from American College of Sports Medicine. *ACSM's Resource Manual for Guidelines for Exercise Testing and Prescription.* 6th ed. Philadelphia (PA): Wolters Kluwer Health Ltd; 2009. 277 p.

ESTIMATION OF GOAL BODY WEIGHT

For those individuals who desire to alter body composition, it is helpful to provide them with an estimation of body weight at a goal body fat percentage. A simple method to derive an estimate of a goal body weight is based on the following equation:

$$\text{Goal body weight} = \text{Fat-free weight}/(1 - [\text{Goal body fat percentage}/100])$$

An example of the calculation of goal body weight for a man who weighs 200 lb with an estimated body fat of 25% and a goal body fat of 15% is as follows:

Determine fat-free weight:

$$\text{Fat-free weight} = \text{Body weight} \cdot ([100 - \text{Body fat percentage}]/100)$$
$$= 200 \cdot ([100 - 25]/100) = 150 \text{ lb}$$

Determine goal body weight:

$$\text{Goal body weight} = 150/(1 - [15/100]) = 176.4 \text{ lb}$$

This approach uses the assumption that all of the weight that is lost is body fat.

SUMMARY

Body composition measurements are performed as part of an HRPF evaluation and also provide important information related to functional status. Although there is not a true gold standard measure of body composition, there are many methods that can provide helpful information.

LABORATORY ACTIVITIES

SKINFOLD ESTIMATION OF BODY FAT PERCENTAGE

Data Collection

Work in groups of three and make all skinfold measurements on every member of your group (one technician, one subject, one recorder). Use *Box 4.2* as a guide for identifying appropriate skinfold sites. Take each measurement twice (take a third if the first two differ by more than 2 mm) and average the two closest measures. Use *Box 4.3* to calculate Db from skinfold measurements and use the Siri equation (9) to calculate fat percentage from Db (when using Db to calculate body fat percentage, carry the Db value out four places past the decimal). Calculate your body fat using the seven-site formula and *each* of the three-site formulas in *Box 4.3*. Show your calculations on a separate sheet of paper and hand them in with the rest of the assignment. Record values obtained on you.

Written Report

1. Using your fat percentage value for the seven-site formula for the first technician, what range of values would represent ±1 SEE unit encompassing 68% of the population with these same fat percentage values?
2. How did the fat percentage values obtained from the seven- and three-site formulas compare for the first technician?
3. How reliable were the two technicians in determining body fat percentage and the skinfold measures at each site?
4. Using the seven-site formula, what is your fat weight from each technician?

5. Using the seven-site formula, what is your fat-free weight from each technician?
6. Compare the body fat percentile to the classification of disease risk based on BMI and waist circumference (see *Table 3.3*). Are these two interpretations consistent?

Technician: _____   Height (in or cm): _____   Weight (lb or kg): _____

	Skinfolds			Mean
Abdominal	____ mm	____ mm	____ mm	= ____ mm
Triceps	____ mm	____ mm	____ mm	= ____ mm
Biceps	____ mm	____ mm	____ mm	= ____ mm
Chest/pectoral	____ mm	____ mm	____ mm	= ____ mm
Midaxillary	____ mm	____ mm	____ mm	= ____ mm
Subscapular	____ mm	____ mm	____ mm	= ____ mm
Suprailiac	____ mm	____ mm	____ mm	= ____ mm
Thigh	____ mm	____ mm	____ mm	= ____ mm
Seven-site formula: ____ % fat				
Three-site formula: ____ % fat				
Three-site formula: ____ % fat				
	Circumference			Mean
Waist	____ cm	____ cm	____ cm	= ____ cm

CASE STUDY

David is a 45-yr-old man who came in to the ABC Fitness Club for a body composition evaluation. David weighed 187 lb and was tested in a whole body plethysmograph. His body volume was determined to be 81.5 L. What is David's estimated body fat percentage, including the SEE? Provide David with an interpretation of his estimated body fat percentage using a percentile score. If David desired to be at the 75th percentile for men his age, what is his goal body weight at that desired level of body fat?

REFERENCES

1. Boren HG, Kory RC, Snyder JC. The Veteran's Administration Army Cooperative study of pulmonary function. II. The lung volume and its subdivisions in normal men. *Am J Med*. 1966;41:96–114.
2. Brozek J, Grade F, Anderson J. Densitometric analysis of body composition: revision of some quantitative assumptions. *Ann N Y Acad Sci*. 1963;110:113–40.
3. Callaway CW, Chumlea WC, Bouchard C, Himes JH, Lohman TG, Martin AD. Circumferences. In: Lohman TG, Roche AF, Martorell R, editors. *Anthropometric Standardization Reference Manual*. Champaign: Human Kinetics; 1988. p. 39–80.
4. Heyward VH, Wagner DR. *Applied Body Composition Assessment*. 2nd ed. Champaign (IL): Human Kinetics; 2004. 268 p.
5. Jackson AS, Pollock ML. Practical assessment of body composition. *Phys Sport Med*. 1985;13:76–90.
6. National Center for Chronic Disease Prevention and Health Promotion, Division of Adolescent and School Health. Healthy youth: Health topics, childhood obesity. *Centers for Disease Control and Prevention* [Internet]. Modified 3 June 2010 [cited 2011 Jul 8]. Available from: http://www.cdc.gov/healthyyouth/obesity/
7. O'Brien RJ, Drizd TA. Roentgenographic determination of total lung capacity: normal values from a national population survey. *Am Rev Respir Dis*. 1983;128:949–52.

8. Pollock ML, Schmidt DH, Jackson AS. Measurement of cardiorespiratory fitness and body composition in the clinical setting. *Comp Ther*. 1980;6:12–7.

9. Siri WE. The gross composition of the body. *Adv Biol Med Physiol*. 1956;4:239–80.

10. Walker, R. Summary: Mass, weight, density or specific gravity of water at various temperatures C and thermal coefficient of expansion of water. *SImetric* [Internet]. Modified 11 Feb 2010 [cited 2011 Jul 8]. Available from: http://www.simetric.co.uk/si_water.htm#tenth

Muscular Fitness

WHY MEASURE MUSCULAR FITNESS?

Muscular fitness is well accepted as an important prerequisite for good physical function. Think of the times the assistance of a strong person is needed to help move a heavy object like a couch, or to unload a large delivery of items like 40-lb bags, for a house project. These are examples of the necessity of muscular fitness. As individuals age, muscular fitness becomes even more important because sarcopenia is clearly an issue for reduced functional abilities and quality of life for senior citizens. Seniors with inadequate muscular fitness may ultimately have difficulty performing routine daily tasks, such as carrying or unloading groceries.

There are also clear health-related reasons to have good muscular fitness. These include improved posture, less risk of musculoskeletal injuries, better bone mass (decreased risk of osteoporosis), improved glucose uptake (better blood glucose control), and potentially increased resting metabolic rate (better body weight control).

Performing a comprehensive muscular fitness assessment presents some challenges and will be time consuming, and this has unfortunately resulted in underutilization of the process in programs that perform health-related physical fitness (HRPF) assessments. It is hoped that this trend will change, as current public health guidelines prominently advocate muscular fitness activities. The *2008 Physical Activity Guidelines for Americans* provided by the U.S. Department of Health and Human Services recommends that "adults should also do muscle-strengthening activities that are moderate or high intensity and involve all major muscle groups on 2 or more days a week, as these activities provide additional health benefits" (8). These guidelines further advocate muscular fitness activities for children, older adults, and even individuals with chronic disease (with appropriate modifications as designated by one's health care provider).

UNIQUE ASSESSMENT PRINCIPLES

Muscular strength and muscular endurance are measurable components of HRPF. One unique aspect of muscle measurements is that there are approximately 700 skeletal muscles in the human body, each of which can yield a different level of performance. So unlike body composition and cardiorespiratory endurance, there is no single measurement that provides an assessment of an individual's muscular strength or muscular endurance. Then, to further complicate the assessment of muscular fitness, there are different types of muscular contractions. Because many muscular contractions involve more than one muscle, performance can vary with technique and variation of the method employed to load the muscle. Each of these factors (type of contraction, familiarization, method of loading, body positioning, and specificity) can influence muscular strength and muscular endurance assessments (1).

TYPES OF CONTRACTIONS

Basically, there are two principal types of muscular contractions: static and dynamic. During a static contraction, the muscle generates force without movement taking place. This may involve pushing or pulling against an immovable object or holding an object in place. These are also called isometric ("iso" meaning equal and "metric" meaning length) contractions because the length of the muscle does not change during the execution of the contraction.

Dynamic contractions are those that generate force to move an object. The muscle changes in length during these contractions. Contractions that occur during the lengthening of a muscle are termed eccentric, whereas those involving muscle shortening are termed concentric. Additionally, if the movement involves a fixed amount of resistance, it is called an isotonic contraction; and if movement takes place at a fixed speed, it is termed an isokinetic contraction. *Chapter 31 of ACSM's Resource Manual for Guidelines for Exercise Testing and Prescription* contains a more thorough overview of factors related to muscular contractions.

FAMILIARIZATION

Some assessment procedures for muscular fitness may require tasks that are uncommon and infrequently performed by the client. Like many other activities, a person's performance can be improved through learning and then practicing a technique. This is often called a learning effect. Thus, many muscular fitness assessments will actually require a period of time to allow the client to learn and become familiar with the procedures. Failure to allow for this familiarization will affect the accuracy of the assessment results.

Client performance is also related to the opportunity for a warm-up period prior to participation in the muscular fitness assessments. Five to 10 min of light intensity aerobic exercise (*e.g.*, treadmill or cycle) is recommended, followed by several low-intensity repetitions of the exercise being tested. Beyond the physiologic factors of increasing blood circulation to the muscles and increasing the temperature of the muscles, a warm-up allows a familiarization refresher immediately prior to the assessment.

METHOD OF LOADING

Free weights and resistance exercise machines are the two major sources of resistance to the muscle for dynamic contractions. Each has advantages and disadvantages, both for assessment and training. Among the advantages for free weights are uniformity (*i.e.*, a 25-lb weight plate is the same at every facility), the wide range of movement patterns that can be performed, and the similarity of movement to everyday activities (*e.g.*, lifting and putting a 25-lb box on an overhead shelf). The disadvantages to free weights for assessment purposes are potential difficulty in isolating a muscle group and safety issues related to dropping the weights.

Resistance exercise machines with supported weights, as shown in *Figure 5.1*, generally can overcome the disadvantages of free weights by limiting a contraction to a specific pattern in an effort to better isolate a muscle group and by minimizing risk to the client from a dropped weight. However, the disadvantages of these machines are that movement patterns are limited to one per machine, these isolated patterns are not necessarily typical of everyday activities, and significant variability can exist in the designated amount of weight between different brands of machines (*e.g.*, some machines only use a 1, 2, 3, 4 . . . system to designate a difference in load vs. actual

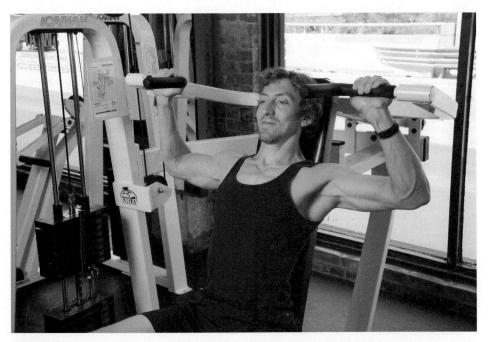

■ **FIGURE 5.1.** An example of a resistance exercise unit that uses a weight stack for loading.

pounds lifted). Also, many machines have some type of mechanism that varies the resistance applied throughout the range of motion of the contraction. Different manufacturers have different mechanisms to vary the resistance (cams, levers, pulleys, etc.). Obviously, this creates difficulties in comparing results from assessments performed on different resistance exercise machines. The ability to track an individual over the course of many years can also be affected if the machines used by a facility are upgraded with new models. This issue can be addressed by performing a comparison check on the old versus the new equipment to determine if any differences may exist. If differences are found, a correction factor can be developed, allowing for more accurate comparisons.

In muscular endurance testing, some of the assessments use an individual's body weight as the source of the resistance. Additionally, some tests employ a fixed amount of absolute weight, whereas others may use a fixed percentage of a person's maximum capacity. Depending on the method used to select the resistance, the outcome will vary.

PROPER POSITIONING

Proper positioning is essential for assessments using either free weights or machines. Standardization of the positioning allows for accurate measurement of the muscle group being assessed. Variations in positioning can potentially allow other muscle groups to contribute to movement of the load, which will increase the amount of weight recorded for the assessment, producing inaccurate results. Also, proper positioning may be necessary for the safety of the client.

SPECIFICITY

The principle of specificity is most typically applied to exercise training where an exercise program has been tailored to precisely mimic a specific performance goal or activity. Specificity also has relevance for assessment because each muscle group tested will have different capabilities depending on the specific requirements of the test methodology. The strength or endurance of a muscle will be specific to the size of the muscle and limb, the type of contraction, the exact movement pattern (or the joint angle for a static measure), the speed of the movement, and the amount of resistance. Because these specificity characteristics vary between different muscular fitness assessment procedures, interpretation of test results becomes challenging. One key for HRPF assessment of muscular fitness is standardization within the measurement procedure.

MUSCULAR FITNESS CONTINUUM

Muscular fitness is a term that encompasses both muscular strength and endurance. From an assessment perspective, strength is the measurement of the maximal force capability of the muscle, and endurance is the measurement of the ability to continue performing contractions at a submaximal level. Muscular fitness is typically viewed on a continuum — a model of overall muscular performance — where pure strength and pure endurance represent polar ends.

STRENGTH ASSESSMENTS

The assessment of muscular strength will be specific to the muscle group and the other unique assessment factors reviewed earlier. Thus, there is no one single measure of muscular strength for an individual. The best case scenario for HRPF assessment of muscular strength would be to use an assessment of a group of different muscles in some sort of composite score to capture a concept of overall strength of an individual. However, even this approach would be limited in the case of a person with excellent strength levels in some muscles and poor strength levels in other muscles, leading to an inaccurate interpretation of average overall muscle strength.

A major decision to be made, which also applies to endurance measurements, involves selecting the method of resistance for the assessments. This decision will be dictated, in part, by the interpretation scale to be used (*i.e.*, if the norms were developed from free weights, then free weights should be used for the assessment).

STATIC

Historically, static measures, with origins in physical education classes, have been used to assess strength. Although grip strength has been widely employed, a variety of different static measures can be performed using either dynamometers or tensiometers. These tests have been popular and widely used in physical education programs owing to their low cost and durability.

Dynamometers

The most commonly performed static strength test is the measurement of grip strength using a handgrip dynamometer. Grip strength norms are given in *Table 5.1*, and the procedures for the grip strength test are described in *Box 5.1* and illustrated in *Figure 5.2*.

Another test that has recently been used in fitness settings is the assessment of static back and leg strength. An example of the type of dynamometer used for this assessment is shown in *Figure 5.3*.

Tensiometers

Another popular form of static strength assessment employs a cable tensiometer. These units can be adjusted to test multiple joint angles through a range of motion for a particular muscular contraction. They can be mounted to walls or tables and set up to

TABLE 5.1. Grip-Strength Norms						
Age (yr)	15–19		20–29		30–39	
Gender	M	F	M	F	M	F
Above average	103–112	64–70	113–123	65–70	113–122	66–72
Average	95–102	59–63	106–112	61–64	105–112	61–65
Below average	84–94	54–58	97–105	55–60	97–104	56–60
Poor	≤83	≤53	≤96	≤54	≤96	≤55
Age (yr)	40–49		50–59		60–69	
Gender	M	F	M	F	M	F
Above average	110–118	65–72	102–109	59–64	98–101	54–59
Average	102–109	59–64	96–101	55–58	86–92	51–53
Below average	94–101	55–58	87–95	51–54	79–85	48–50
Poor	≤93	≤54	≤86	≤50	≤78	≤47

Reprinted with permission from the Canadian Society for Exercise Physiology. *Canadian Physical Activity, Fitness & Lifestyle Approach: CSEP-Health & Fitness Program's Health-Related Appraisal & Counseling Strategy.* 3rd ed. Ottawa (Canada): Canadian Society for Exercise Physiology; 2003. 300 p.

BOX 5.1	Procedures for the Static Handgrip Strength Test

1. Have the client stand for the test. Usually, this test is performed with each hand. The norms provided use a combined score for the right and left hands. The test can also be performed with only the dominant hand.
2. Adjust the grip bar so that the second joint of the fingers will be bent to grip the handle of the dynamometer.
3. Have the client hold the handgrip dynamometer parallel to the side of the body. The elbow should be flexed at 90 degrees. Make sure that the dynamometer is set to zero.
4. The client should then squeeze the handgrip dynamometer as hard as possible without holding the breath (to avoid the Valsalva maneuver). It is optional if the client wishes to extend the elbow; however, other body movement should be avoided.
5. Record the grip strength in kilograms. Repeat this procedure using the opposite hand.
6. Repeat the test two more times with each hand. Take the highest of the three readings for each hand and add these two values (one from each hand) together as the measure of handgrip strength to compare with the norms presented in *Table 5.1*.

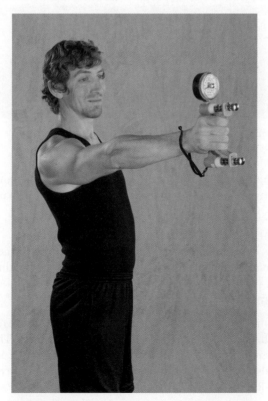

■ **FIGURE 5.2.** Measurement of static strength with a handgrip dynamometer.

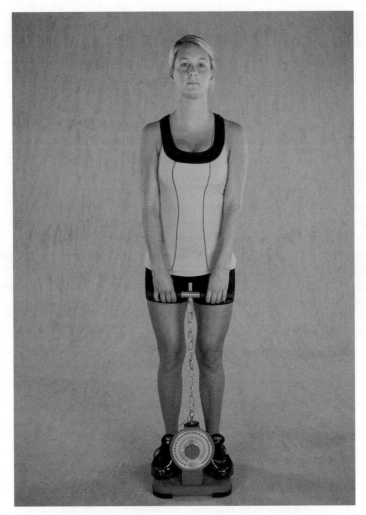

■ **FIGURE 5.3.** Measurement of back strength with a dynamometer.

mimic various common activities. These were more popular in sports-related physical fitness and therefore will not be discussed in more detail in this manual.

DYNAMIC

As reviewed earlier, dynamic muscular contractions can be performed with either concentric or eccentric movements and with different methods of loading the resistance.

Repetition Maximum

Repetition maximum (RM) is the term used to describe the maximal amount of weight that can be lifted through a full range of motion with good form. The one RM (1-RM) is typically considered as the gold standard measure of muscular strength (5). Some fitness professionals have developed strength assessment protocols using multiple repetitions (*e.g.,* 4-RM, 6-RM, 8-RM). Although there are no clear standards or norms available for these evaluations, there are some equations to predict a 1-RM value from these multiple-RM tests (3).

BOX 5.2	Procedures for a One Repetition Maximum (1-RM) Assessment (7)

1. The subject should warm up by completing several submaximal repetitions.
2. Determine the 1-RM (or any multiple-RM) within four trials with rest periods of 3–5 min between trials.
3. Select an initial weight that is within the subject's perceived capacity (~50%–70% of capacity).
4. Progressively increase resistance by 2.5–20 kg until the subject cannot complete the selected repetition(s); all repetitions should be performed at the same speed of movement and range of motion to ensure consistency between trials.
5. Record the final weight lifted successfully as the absolute 1-RM or multiple-RM.

American College of Sports Medicine. Health-related physical fitness testing and interpretation. In: *ACSM's Guidelines for Exercise Testing and Prescription*. 9th ed. Philadelphia: Wolters Kluwer Health Ltd; 2011. 480 p.

The 1-RM test can be performed with any muscle group and can be tested using either free weights or machines. The procedures for performing a 1-RM assessment are provided in *Box 5.2*. It is quite common in HRPF assessments to use the bench press as a general measure of upper body strength and the leg press for lower body strength. *Tables 5.2* and *5.3* provide normative reference data for these two tests.

Isokinetic

Isokinetic (contraction at a constant velocity) assessments of muscular fitness require specialized and expensive equipment. The assessments can include a wide range of data (*e.g.*, maximal tension throughout a complete range of motion) that prove highly reliable and accurate. These tests are commonly performed in both athletic and physical therapy rehabilitative programs. However, because of the expense of the equipment and the relatively long time period required to complete an assessment of one muscle group, this type of assessment is not commonly performed in HRPF assessment programs.

ENDURANCE ASSESSMENTS

Like muscular strength assessment, the assessment of muscular endurance will be specific to the muscle group and the other unique assessment factors reviewed earlier. Endurance assessments can be conducted by performing a fixed amount of contractions in a defined time period, by performing a maximal number of contractions of a set resistance, or by holding a static contraction for a period of time.

DYNAMIC

Dynamic tests of muscular endurance can be performed with free weights or resistance exercise machines. Additionally, these tests can be performed using calisthenic-type exercises, which were popular in physical education classes. This section will cover some of the more common endurance tests that have been used, which have normative values for interpretation. However, fitness professionals often create their own tests and can use these as serial assessments over time with a client.

TABLE 5.2. Fitness Categories for Upper Body Strength[a] for Men and Women by Age

Bench Press Weight Ratio $= \dfrac{\text{weight pushed in lbs}}{\text{body weight in lbs}}$

MEN						
		Age				
%		**<20**	**20–29**	**30–39**	**40–49**	**50–59**	**60+**
99	Superior	>1.76	>1.63	>1.35	>1.20	>1.05	>0.94
95		1.76	1.63	1.35	1.20	1.05	0.94
90	Excellent	1.46	1.48	1.24	1.10	0.97	0.89
85		1.38	1.37	1.17	1.04	0.93	0.84
80		1.34	1.32	1.12	1.00	0.90	0.82
75	Good	1.29	1.26	1.08	0.96	0.87	0.79
70		1.24	1.22	1.04	0.93	0.84	0.77
65		1.23	1.18	1.01	0.90	0.81	0.74
60		1.19	1.14	0.98	0.88	0.79	0.72
55	Fair	1.16	1.10	0.96	0.86	0.77	0.70
50		1.13	1.06	0.93	0.84	0.75	0.68
45		1.10	1.03	0.90	0.82	0.73	0.67
40		1.06	0.99	0.88	0.80	0.71	0.66
35	Poor	1.01	0.96	0.86	0.78	0.70	0.65
30		0.96	0.93	0.83	0.76	0.68	0.63
25		0.93	0.90	0.81	0.74	0.66	0.60
20		0.89	0.88	0.78	0.72	0.63	0.57
15	Very poor	0.86	0.84	0.75	0.69	0.60	0.56
10		0.81	0.80	0.71	0.65	0.57	0.53
5		0.76	0.72	0.65	0.59	0.53	0.49
1		<0.76	<0.72	<0.65	<0.59	<0.53	<0.49
n		60	425	1,909	2,090	1,279	343

Total $n = 6,106$

WOMEN						
99	Superior	>0.88	>1.01	>0.82	>0.77	>0.68	>0.72
95		0.88	1.01	0.82	0.77	0.68	0.72
90	Excellent	0.83	0.90	0.76	0.71	0.61	0.64
85		0.81	0.83	0.72	0.66	0.57	0.59
80		0.77	0.80	0.70	0.62	0.55	0.54
75	Good	0.76	0.77	0.65	0.60	0.53	0.53
70		0.74	0.74	0.63	0.57	0.52	0.51
65		0.70	0.72	0.62	0.55	0.50	0.48
60		0.65	0.70	0.60	0.54	0.48	0.47
55	Fair	0.64	0.68	0.58	0.53	0.47	0.46
50		0.63	0.65	0.57	0.52	0.46	0.45
45		0.60	0.63	0.55	0.51	0.45	0.44
40		0.58	0.59	0.53	0.50	0.44	0.43

(continued)

TABLE 5.2. Fitness Categories for Upper Body Strength[a] for Men and Women by Age (Continued)

Bench Press Weight Ratio = $\dfrac{\text{weight pushed in lbs}}{\text{body weight in lbs}}$

			WOMEN			
				Age		
%		<20	20–29	30–39	40–49	50–59	60+
35		0.57	0.58	0.52	0.48	0.43	0.41
30	Poor	0.56	0.56	0.51	0.47	0.42	0.40
25		0.55	0.53	0.49	0.45	0.41	0.39
20		0.53	0.51	0.47	0.43	0.39	0.38
15		0.52	0.50	0.45	0.42	0.38	0.36
10	Very poor	0.50	0.48	0.42	0.38	0.37	0.33
5		0.41	0.44	0.39	0.35	0.31	0.26
1		<0.41	<0.44	<0.39	<0.35	<0.31	<0.26
n		20	191	379	333	189	42

Total n = 1,154

[a]One repetition maximum bench press, with bench press weight ratio = weight pushed in pounds per body weight in pounds.

Adapted with permission from *Physical Fitness Assessments and Norms for Adults and Law Enforcement*. The Cooper Institute, Dallas, Texas. 2009. For more information: www.cooperinstitute.org

TABLE 5.3. Fitness Categories for Leg Strength by Age and Sex[a]

Percentile		Age (year)				
		20–29	30–39	40–49	50–59	60+
		Men				
90	Well above average	2.27	2.07	1.92	1.80	1.73
80	Above average	2.13	1.93	1.82	1.71	1.62
70		2.05	1.85	1.74	1.64	1.56
60	Average	1.97	1.77	1.68	1.58	1.49
50		1.91	1.71	1.62	1.52	1.43
40	Below average	1.83	1.65	1.57	1.46	1.38
30		1.74	1.59	1.51	1.39	1.30
20	Well below average	1.63	1.52	1.44	1.32	1.25
10		1.51	1.43	1.35	1.22	1.16
		Women				
90	Well above average	1.82	1.61	1.48	1.37	1.32
80	Above average	1.68	1.47	1.37	1.25	1.18
70		1.58	1.39	1.29	1.17	1.13
60	Average	1.50	1.33	1.23	1.10	1.04
50		1.44	1.27	1.18	1.05	0.99
40	Below average	1.37	1.21	1.13	0.99	0.93
30		1.27	1.15	1.08	0.95	0.88
20	Well below average	1.22	1.09	1.02	0.88	0.85
10		1.14	1.00	0.94	0.78	0.72

[a]One repetition maximum leg press with leg press weight ratio = weight pushed per body weight.

Adapted from Institute for Aerobics Research, Dallas, 1994. Study population for the data set was predominantly white and college educated. A Universal Dynamic Variable Resistance (DVR) machine was used to measure the 1-repetition maximum (RM).

BOX 5.3	Procedures for the YMCA Submaximal Bench Press Test (6)

The test requires a 35-lb bar for women and a bar with weights totaling 80 lb for men.

1. Position the client on the bench (supine position) with both feet on the floor.
2. A spotter should hand the barbell to the client (hands shoulder width apart) and be available throughout the test to grasp the barbell when necessary. The test is started in the down position with the bar touching the chest.
3. Set a metronome to 60 beats per minute and have the client perform a contraction by lifting the bar to full extension with one beat and then lowering the bar to touch the chest with the next beat. The lifting cadence will produce 30 repetitions per minute. Encourage the client to breathe regularly to avoid the Valsalva maneuver.
4. The test continues until the client is unable to reach full extention of elbows or cannot complete a repetition on schedule with the cadence while using correct form. (Note: For highly fit subjects, an upper limit may need to be established.)

Results are compared with the norms presented in *Table 5.4.*

YMCA Submaximal Bench Press Test

This test provides a standardized method to quantify muscular endurance using the bench press exercise. The procedures for this test are provided in *Box 5.3* and interpretative norms are located in *Table 5.4.* Other variations of this test that are sometimes used assess the number of repetitions a person can perform at a certain percentage of his or her 1-RM or body weight (*e.g.*, 70%).

TABLE 5.4. Fitness Categories for the YMCA Bench Press Test (Total Lifts) by Age and Sex

Category	Age (year)											
	18–25		26–35		36–45		46–55		56–65		>65	
Sex	M	W	M	W	M	W	M	W	M	W	M	W
Excellent	64	66	61	62	55	57	47	50	41	42	36	30
	44	42	41	40	36	33	28	29	24	24	20	18
Good	41	38	37	34	32	30	25	24	21	21	16	16
	34	30	30	29	26	26	21	20	17	17	12	12
Above average	33	28	29	28	25	24	20	18	14	14	10	10
	29	25	26	24	22	21	16	14	12	12	9	8
Average	28	22	24	22	21	20	14	13	11	10	8	7
	24	20	21	18	18	16	12	10	9	8	7	5
Below average	22	18	20	17	17	14	11	9	8	6	6	4
	20	16	17	14	14	12	9	7	5	5	4	3
Poor	17	13	16	13	12	10	8	6	4	4	3	2
	13	9	12	9	9	6	5	2	2	2	2	0
Very poor	<10	6	9	6	6	4	2	1	1	1	1	0

M, men; W, women.

Field Tests

Field tests are particularly useful when testing a large number of people at one time, which is one reason they became popular in physical education classes. Additionally, these tests do not require any equipment and thus can be performed in many different locations, including at home. The two most common field tests are the push-up test and the curl-up test. There are different procedural options (see *Fig. 5.4* for an example) available for the test, some of which count the number of repetitions completed in a fixed period of time. It is important to follow the procedures used to establish the normative values that will be used for interpretation. The procedures for the push-up test are provided in *Box 5.4*, and those for the curl-up test are displayed in *Box 5.5*. Normative data for interpretation of test results are found in *Tables 5.5* and *5.6*.

STATIC

Another option for muscular endurance assessment is the use of timed tests of holding a submaximal contraction. Some versions of these tests can be created by fitness professionals and used in serial assessments over time with a client. One standardized version of a static muscular endurance test is the timed flexed arm hang. The procedures for this test are provided in *Box 5.6*. Some organizations (President's Challenge and U.S. Marine Corps.) have standards for rating either students or military personnel; however, true national norms are lacking.

INTERPRETATION ISSUES

There are several issues that complicate the interpretation of results of muscular fitness assessments. Several confounding factors accompany this unique assessment, including different types of contractions for each muscle, the possibility of a learning curve, improper positioning or incorrect form to allow accessory muscles to contribute to the force, and differences between various methods of loading the resistance. Owing to these multiple factors, a standardized assessment of muscular strength and/or muscular endurance has not been developed.

This chapter provides a variety of different assessment procedures that have been used for many years and for which some normative data exist. These normative data allow for interpretation of the muscular strength and muscular endurance of certain muscles. When using these tables of normative data, it is critical to follow the standardized procedures, which includes using the same equipment as was used by the population from which the norms were developed. This may be difficult when resistance exercise machines are used to develop the normative chart. A case in point is found with *Table 5.3*, which provides data for the leg press. These data were developed using the cohort from the Cooper Clinic, which is a large data set from the population tested at this popular center in Dallas, Texas. The data were originally derived from assessments performed using the universal Dynamic Variable Resistance (DVR) multistation resistance machines, which were widely available for a period of time. However, as the manufacturers of resistance exercise machines developed newer equipment, these universal machines were phased out and are no longer available for purchase. This leads to a dilemma when comparing and assessing clients tested with free weights or other brands of resistance exercise machines. Although the American College of Sports Medicine (ACSM) continues to use this as the primary interpretation chart for this test with the presumption that the weight-press ratio will be similar using other equipment, caution must be exercised because this has not been objectively validated.

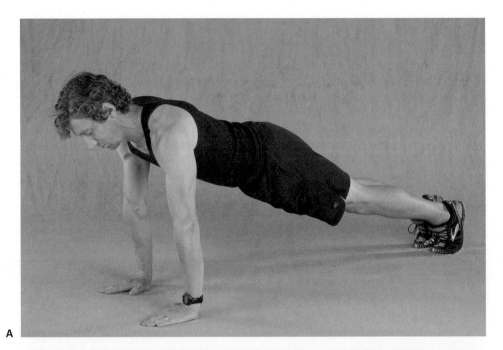

A

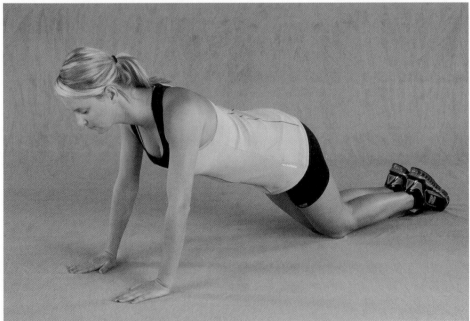

B

■ **FIGURE 5.4.** Different starting positions for men **(A)** and women **(B)** for the push-up test.

BOX 5.4   Push-up Test Procedures for Measurement of Muscular Endurance

PUSH-UP

1. The push-up test is administered with male subjects starting in the standard "down" position (hands pointing forward and under the shoulder, back straight, head up, using the toes as the pivotal point) and female subjects in the modified "knee push-up" position (legs together, lower leg in contact with mat with ankles plantar-flexed, back straight, hands shoulder width apart, head up, using the knees as the pivotal point).
2. The subject must raise the body by straightening the elbows and return to the "down" position, until the chin touches the mat. The stomach should not touch the mat.
3. For both men and women, the subject's back must be straight at all times and the subject must push up to a straight arm position.
4. The maximal number of push-ups performed consecutively without rest is counted as the score.
5. The test is stopped when the client strains forcibly or is unable to maintain the appropriate technique within two repetitions.

Reprinted with permission from the Canadian Society for Exercise Physiology. *Canadian Physical Activity, Fitness & Lifestyle Approach: CSEP-Health & Fitness Program's Health-Related Appraisal & Counseling Strategy.* 3rd ed. Ottawa (Canada): Canadian Society for Exercise Physiology; 2003. 300 p.

BOX 5.5   Curl-up (Crunch) Test Procedures for Measurement of Muscular Endurance

CURL-UP (CRUNCH)

1. The individual assumes a supine position on a mat with the knees at 90 degrees. The arms are at the side, palms facing down with the middle fingers touching a piece of masking tape. A second piece of masking tape is placed 10 cm apart.[a] Shoes remain on during the test.
2. A metronome is set to 50 beats · min[-1] and the individual does slow, controlled curl-ups to lift the shoulder blades off the mat (trunk makes a 30-degree angle with the mat) in time with the metronome at a rate of 25 per minute. The test is done for 1 minute. The low back should be flattened before curling up.
3. Individual performs as many curl-ups as possible without pausing, to a maximum of 25.[b]

[a]Alternatives include (a) having the hands held across the chest, with the head activating a counter when the trunk reaches a 30-degree position (2) and placing the hands on the thighs and curling up until the hands reach the knee caps (4). Elevation of the trunk to 30 degrees is the important aspect of the movement.
[b]An alternative includes doing as many curl-ups as possible in 1 minute.
Reprinted with permission from the Canadian Society for Exercise Physiology. *Canadian Physical Activity, Fitness & Lifestyle Approach: CSEP-Health & Fitness Program's Health-Related Appraisal & Counseling Strategy.* 3rd ed. Ottawa (Canada): Canadian Society for Exercise Physiology; 2003. 300 p.

TABLE 5.5. Fitness Categories for Push-up

Category		Age								
		20–29		30–39		40–49		50–59		60–69	
Sex		M	F	M	F	M	F	M	F	M	F
Excellent		36	30	30	27	25	24	21	21	18	17
Very good		35	29	29	26	24	23	20	20	17	16
		29	21	22	20	17	15	13	11	11	12
Good		28	20	21	19	16	14	12	10	10	11
		22	15	17	13	13	11	10	7	8	5
Fair		21	14	16	12	12	10	9	6	7	4
		17	10	12	8	10	5	7	2	5	2
Needs improvement		16	9	11	7	9	4	6	1	4	1

Reprinted with permission from the Canadian Society for Exercise Physiology. *Canadian Physical Activity, Fitness & Lifestyle Approach: CSEP-Health & Fitness Program's Health-Related Appraisal & Counseling Strategy.* 3rd ed. Ottawa (Canada): Canadian Society for Exercise Physiology; 2003. 300 p.

TABLE 5.6. Fitness Categories for the Partial Curl-Up by Age and Sex

Percentile		Age (year)									
		20–29		30–39		40–49		50–59		60–69	
Gender		M	W	M	W	M	W	M	W	M	W
90	Well above average	75	70	75	55	75	55	74	48	53	50
80	Above average	56	45	69	43	75	42	60	30	33	30
70		41	37	46	34	67	33	45	23	26	24
60	Average	31	32	36	28	51	28	35	16	19	19
50		27	27	31	21	39	25	27	9	16	13
40	Below average	24	21	26	15	31	20	23	2	9	9
30		20	17	19	12	26	14	19	0	6	3
20	Well below average	13	12	13	0	21	5	13	0	0	0
10		4	5	0	0	13	0	0	0	0	0

M, men; W, women.
Adapted from (4).

BOX 5.6   Procedures for the Flexed-Arm Hang Test

1. The client stands on a movable box positioned beneath the bar and grasps the bar with an overhand grip (palms facing away) in a position in which the chin is above the bar, elbows are flexed, and the chest is next to the bar.
2. With the client grasping the bar, the box is slid away and a stopwatch is started.
3. The position is held as long as possible.
4. The time is stopped when the chin touches the bar and dips below the bar or the head tilts back to keep the chin above the bar.

Another debated issue is whether to use absolute amounts of weight lifted or to make the amount of weight lifted a proportion of the client's body weight. The norms developed for the bench press and leg press use the ratio method for interpreting results.

Owing to the limitations in having acceptable norms for interpretation, many fitness professionals forego the process of trying to provide a baseline test interpretation. Instead, the baseline data is only used as a reference point for an individual client, for which future assessments will be compared. Obviously, this does not allow an individual to know how he or she compares to others in the same age group or to a criterion-referenced standard. Hopefully, with the national recommendations to incorporate resistance exercise into all adults' exercise programs, the development of a national testing battery with interpretation standards for muscular fitness will follow.

SUMMARY

There are several unique factors that do not allow for one single measurement to be made to determine either muscular strength or muscular endurance. There are, however, several established tests for the assessment of muscular fitness. The importance of this component of HRPF is growing with the increased emphasis on muscular fitness throughout the lifespan.

LABORATORY ACTIVITIES

ASSESSMENT OF MUSCULAR STRENGTH

Data Collection
Work in groups of two or three. If you are working in a group of three, one person will be the subject, another the technician, and another the recorder. Rotate responsibilities until each person has had a chance to serve in each role. Collect the following data on one other member in your group. Record your values on your data sheet.

Handgrip dynamometer (kg):

	Right	Left
Trial 1:	_____	_____
Trial 2:	_____	_____
Trial 3:	_____	_____
Best Score:	_____	_____
Rating (Table 5.1):	_____	

Sum: _____

Upper body strength:

1-RM (lb): _____
Body weight (lb): _____
Bench press/weight ratio: _____
Percentile ranking (Table 5.2): _____

Lower body strength:

1-RM (lb): _____
Leg press/weight ratio: _____
Percentile ranking (Table 5.3): _____

Laboratory Report

A. Describe your overall muscular strength based on these three measurements. Explain any limitations that apply to making this interpretation of overall muscular strength.

B. Locate a different set of norms for these three tests. How do the interpretations differ between the norms from the tables in this manual and the ones you found? Be sure to include the reference for the other set of norms.

MUSCULAR ENDURANCE ASSESSMENT

Data Collection

Work in groups of two or three. If you are working in a group of three, one person will be the subject, another the technician, and another the recorder. Rotate responsibilities until each person has had a chance to serve in each role. Collect the following data on one other member in your group. Record your values on your data sheet.

Curl-ups:

Number of curl-ups (max = 25): _____
Percentile ranking (*Table 5.6*): _____

Push-ups:

Number of push-ups: _____
Percentile ranking (*Table 5.5*): _____

YMCA bench press test:

Number of repetitions: _____
Percentile ranking (*Table 5.4*): _____

Laboratory Report

A. Describe your overall muscular endurance based on these three measurements. Explain any limitations that apply to making this interpretation of overall muscular endurance.

B. Locate a different set of norms for these three tests. How do the interpretations differ between the norms from the tables in this manual and the ones you found? Be sure to include the reference for the other set of norms.

CASE STUDY

Bob, who weighs 175 lb, and Tom, who weighs 225 lb, have become weightlifting partners and have been training together for the past 6 mo. Bob is 33 yr old and Tom is 28 yr old. They both completed strength assessments of 1-RM for the bench press and were able to lift 200 lb on the bench press, whereas Tom lifted 400 lb on the leg press compared to Bob's 350-lb leg press performance. Discuss how you would compare and interpret Bob and Tom's muscular strength.

REFERENCES

1. American College of Sports Medicine. Position stand on progression models in resistance training for healthy adults. *Med Sci Sports Exerc*. 2002;34(2):364–80.
2. Diener MH, Golding LA, Diener D. Validity and reliability of a one-minute half sit-up test of abdominal muscle strength and endurance. *Sports Med Training Rehab*. 1995;6:5–119.

3. Dohoney P, Chromia JA, Lemire D, et al. Prediction of one repetition maximum (1-RM) strength from a 4–6 RM and 7–10 RM submaximal strength test in healthy young adult males. *J Exerc Physiol Online*. 2002;5:54–9.

4. Faulkner RA, Sprigings EJ, McQuarrie A, et al. A partial curl-up protocol for adults based on an analysis of two procedures. *Can J Sports Sci*. 1989;14:135–41.

5. Fernandez R. One repetition maximum clarified. *J Orthop Sports PhysTher*. 2001;31:264.

6. Golding LA, editor. *YMCA Fitness Testing and Assessment Manual*. 4th ed. Champaign (IL): Human Kinetics; 2000. 247 p.

7. Logan P, Fornasiero D, Abernathy P. Protocols for the assessment of isoinertial strength. In: Fore CJ, editor. *Physiological Tests for Elite Athletes*. Champaign: Human Kinetics; 2000. p. 200–21.

8. U.S. Department of Health and Human Services. *2008 Physical Activity Guidelines for Americans*. ODPHP publication U0036 [Internet]. 2008 [cited 2011 Jul 10]. Available from: www.health.gov/paguidelines

9. YMCA of the USA, Golding LA. *YMCA Fitness Testing and Assessment Manual*. 4th ed. Champaign (IL): Human Kinetics; 2000.

FLEXIBILITY AS A COMPONENT OF HEALTH-RELATED PHYSICAL FITNESS

Flexibility assessment is an important component of health-related physical fitness (HRPF) because inadequate flexibility decreases performance of activities of daily living. Additionally, poor lower back and hip flexibility may contribute to the development of lower back pain, which is one of the more costly medical issues faced by many adults.

Determining flexibility of specific joints yields valuable information to an overall HRPF assessment. As with other HRPF measures, flexibility measures are useful as baseline measures to allow comparison of changes following a training program or serially over time as one ages. These baseline and periodic assessments can also identify joints with below desirable levels of flexibility, which can then be targeted for improvement in exercise training programs. Additionally, these assessments may help in identifying bilateral strength imbalances in the muscles functioning about the joint. When assessing joint range of motion (ROM), bilateral comparison can identify differences in ROM between the left and right structures being evaluated. ROM deviations may lead to muscle imbalances and cause adjacent joint and muscle structures to overcompensate within the kinetic chain of movement, resulting in dysfunction within the related joint structures and the potential to develop injuries, trauma, and movement pattern complications.

UNIQUE ASSESSMENT PRINCIPLES

Flexibility is the functional capacity of the joints to move through a full ROM. The gold standard for determining flexibility is the laboratory assessment of the ROM of a specific joint. As was the case for muscular fitness, there are literally hundreds of joints in the human body, each of which can have a different level of flexibility. Indeed, entire manuals have been devoted to assessment of ROM of the human body joints (3,6). Two requirements of any flexibility assessment are that it be specific to a joint and that an adequate warm-up is provided for the client.

SPECIFICITY

Flexibility is joint specific and therefore will vary depending on which muscle and joint are being evaluated. This essentially rules out the possibility of a single test that can truly characterize one's flexibility. Additionally, each joint has a set ROM that is unique to the function of the specific joint.

WARM-UP

An adequate warm-up is essential prior to assessing flexibility. The warm-up should begin with some whole-body aerobic exercise such as walking or cycling as depicted in *Figure 6.1.* Ideally, both arms and legs should be involved to increase blood flow and temperature. Some passive stretching and ROM exercises of the joints to be assessed should then follow the aerobic warm-up.

METHODS OF MEASUREMENT

Many different methods are used for assessing flexibility. These range from fairly simple visual methods, to measuring the change in reach distance, to using specially designed devices to assess ROM, including new technology that uses digital video cameras and software. The most widely used device for determining ROM is a goniometer, with some such instruments using an electronic scale (electrogoniometers). The goniometer measurement of joint movement in degrees is considered the gold standard measure for flexibility assessment. Other devices for flexibility assessment include the Leighton flexometer and inclinometers.

This manual will focus on the assessment of some of the major joints in the body that are used to perform physical activities and exercise for health-related reasons. Assessments made both with measures of reach distance and with a goniometer will be reviewed.

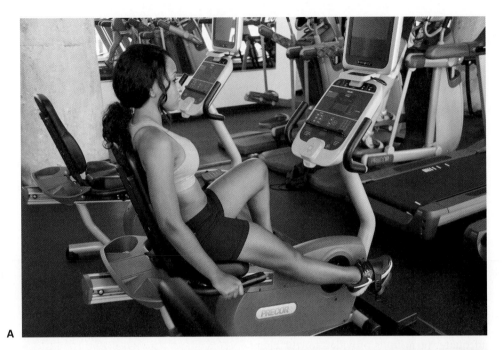

A

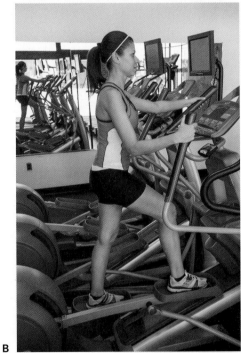

B

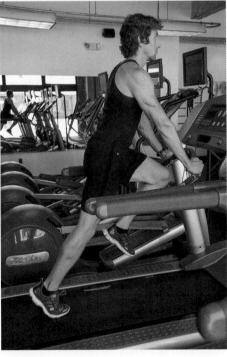

C

■ **FIGURE 6.1.** A flexibility assessment should be preceded by a warm-up period that could include cycling **(A)**, ellipitical trainers **(B)**, or walking or jogging on a treadmill **(C)**.

DISTANCE TESTS FOR ASSESSMENT OF FLEXIBILITY

SIT-AND-REACH TEST

Probably the most widely used flexibility test in physical fitness programs is the sit-and-reach test. This test became popular based on the belief that limitations in this bending and reaching movement are associated with low back pain and may predispose one to a low back injury. It is generally hypothesized that poor abdominal strength and endurance and poor hamstring flexibility are contributing factors to the development of low back pain. The sit-and-reach test provides an assessment of the flexibility of the hamstrings; however, as stated in *ACSM's Guidelines for Exercise Testing and Prescription* (*GETP9*), "its relationship to predict the incidence of low back pain is limited" (5). Thus, it is important not to promote this test as a screening tool for low back issues. Rather, it is a good test for hamstring, hip, and low back flexibility, which are important for many daily activities. The procedures for this test are provided in *Box 6.1*. It should be noted that there are various modifications that have been proposed for the sit-and-reach test; however, norms for all these variations are not well established.

BOX 6.1   Trunk Flexion (Sit-and-Reach) Test Procedures

Pretest: Clients/Patients should perform a short warm-up prior to this test and include some stretches (*e.g.*, modified hurdler's stretch). It is also recommended that the participant refrain from fast, jerky movements, which may increase the possibility of an injury. The participant's shoes should be removed.

1. For the Canadian Trunk Forward Flexion test, the client sits without shoes and the soles of the feet flat against the flexometer (sit-and-reach box) at the 26 cm mark. Inner edges of the soles are placed within 2 cm of the measuring scale. For the YMCA sit-and-reach test, a yardstick is placed on the floor and tape is placed across it at a right angle to the 15 in mark. The client/patient sits with the yardstick between the legs, with legs extended at right angles to the taped line on the floor. Heels of the feet should touch the edge of the taped line and be about 10 to 12 in apart. (Note the zero point at the foot/box interface and use the appropriate norms.)
2. The client/patient should slowly reach forward with both hands as far as possible, holding this position approximately 2 s. Be sure that the participant keeps the hands parallel and does not lead with one hand. Fingertips can be overlapped and should be in contact with the measuring portion or yardstick of the sit-and-reach box.
3. The score is the most distant point (cm or in) reached with the fingertips. The best of two trials should be recorded. To assist with the best attempt, the client/patient should exhale and drop the head between the arms when reaching. Testers should ensure that the knees of the participant stay extended; however, the participant's knees should not be pressed down. The client/patient should breathe normally during the test and should not hold her/his breath at any time. Norms for the Canadian test are presented in *Table 6.1*. Note that these norms use a sit-and-reach box in which the "zero" point is set at the 26 cm mark. If a box is used in which the zero point is set at 23 cm (*e.g.*, Fitnessgram), subtract 3 cm from each value in this table. The norms for the YMCA test are presented in *Table 6.2*.

Reprinted with permission from (2) and (8).

TABLE 6.1. Fitness Categories for Trunk Forward Flexion Using a Sit-and-Reach Box (cm)[a] by Age and Sex

Category		20–29		30–39		40–49		50–59		60–69	
Sex		M	W	M	W	M	W	M	W	M	W
Excellent		40	41	38	41	35	38	35	39	33	35
Very good		39	40	37	40	34	37	34	38	32	34
		34	37	33	36	29	34	28	33	25	31
Good		33	36	32	35	28	33	27	32	24	30
		30	33	28	32	24	30	24	30	20	27
Fair		29	32	27	31	23	29	23	29	19	26
		25	28	23	27	18	25	16	25	15	23
Needs improvement		24	27	22	26	17	24	15	24	14	22

[a]These norms are based on a sit-and-reach box in which the "zero" point is set at 26 cm. When using a box in which the zero point is set at 23 cm, subtract 3 cm from each value in this table.

M, men; W, women.

Reprinted with permission from (2). ©2003. Used with permission from the Canadian Society for Exercise Physiology www.csep.ca

ASSESSMENT OF LUMBAR FLEXION

The lumbar flexion test takes place with the client seated on the floor or table with legs extended and pelvis stabilized to prevent anterior/posterior tilting, as depicted in *Figure 6.2*. Tape is positioned with the zero mark at the spinous process C7, and measurement is taken down to the superior iliac (or level to the posterior superior iliac spine). The client performs lumbar flexion until the first sign of resistance, and the increase in distance is recorded. An average range for healthy adults is a 4-in increase as the spine flexes.

ASSESSMENT OF LUMBAR EXTENSION

The test takes place with the client seated in the same position as was used for lumbar flexion, with the tape positioned in the same starting position, as illustrated in *Figure 6.3*.

TABLE 6.2. Fitness Categories for the YMCA Sit-and-Reach Test (in) by Age and Sex

Percentile		18–25		26–35		36–45		46–55		56–65		>65	
Gender		M	W	M	W	M	W	M	W	M	W	M	W
90	Well above average	22	24	21	23	21	22	19	21	17	20	17	20
80	Above average	20	22	19	21	19	21	17	20	15	19	15	18
70		19	21	17	20	17	19	15	18	13	17	13	17
60	Average	18	20	17	20	16	18	14	17	13	16	12	17
50		17	19	15	19	15	17	13	16	11	15	10	15
40	Below average	15	18	14	17	13	16	11	14	9	14	9	14
30		14	17	13	16	13	15	10	14	9	13	8	13
20	Well below average	13	16	11	15	11	14	9	12	7	11	7	11
10		11	14	9	13	7	12	6	10	5	9	4	9

M, men; W, women.

Adapted with permission from (8). © 2000 by YMCA of the USA, Chicago. All rights reserved.

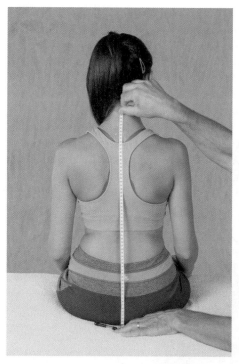

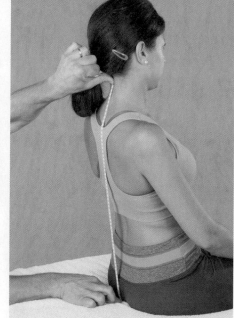

■ FIGURE 6.2. Assessment of lumbar flexion.

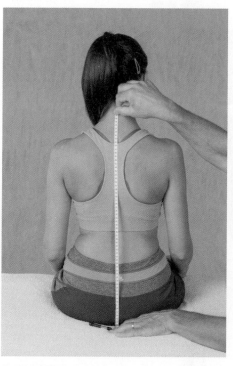

■ FIGURE 6.3. Assessment of lumbar extension.

The client performs lumbar extension until the first sign of resistance. An average range for healthy adults is a 2-in increase as the spine extends (Note: The measuring tape must be in contact with the client's spine for this measure).

RANGE OF MOTION DEFINED

Many of the joints of the body can perform several different kinds of movements, in different planes and at different angles, depending on the type of joint structure and its designated function (1). ROM is defined as the amount of available motion, or arc of motion, that occurs at a specific joint (6). All ROM assessments start in the anatomic start position, except motions in rotation. In the anatomic start position, the body is set at 0 degrees of flexion, extension, abduction, and adduction, as displayed in *Figure 6.4*. ROM can be assessed in two ways: active ROM, which is the motion achieved by

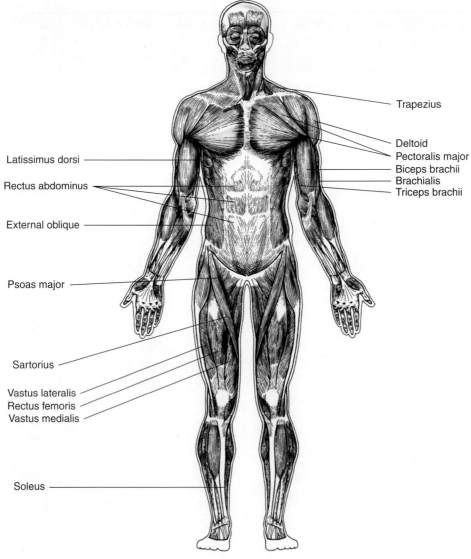

Trapezius

Deltoid
Pectoralis major
Biceps brachii
Brachialis
Triceps brachii

Latissimus dorsi

Rectus abdominus

External oblique

Psoas major

Sartorius

Vastus lateralis
Rectus femoris
Vastus medialis

Soleus

■ **FIGURE 6.4.** Anatomic start position.

the client without assistance by an examiner; or passive ROM, which is the motion achieved by an examiner without the assistance from the client. For HRPF assessments, only active ROM exercises are performed. Passive ROM should only be performed by physicians and allied health professionals such as physical therapists, athletic trainers, and kinesiotherapists, for specific types of medical evaluations.

The fitness professional should be aware of several key factors known to influence flexibility in adults. Age (flexibility tends to decrease with age), gender (flexibility of specific joints is different), previous injuries to the joint (if structural damage occurred or if a surgical procedure was needed), and specific diseases that affect the joint (*e.g.*, arthritis) are all factors that may impact flexibility.

GONIOMETERS — TOOLS TO MEASURE RANGE OF MOTION

The goniometer comes in many different shapes (0–180 degrees or 0–360 degrees), sizes (length of the arms), and materials (metal or plastic). The design of the goniometer, as seen in *Figure 6.5*, includes a body, a fulcrum or center point, a stabilization arm, and a movement arm. The body of a goniometer is similar to a protractor and consists of the arc of a circle. Around the circle are degree measurements that will range from either 0 to 180 degrees or from 0 to 360 degrees. The fulcrum is centered to the identified anatomic landmark required for a given ROM assessment. The stabilization arm is the body segment of the goniometer that will remain fixed and stable during the test. The stabilization arm establishes the starting position of the measurement. The movement arm is the body segment of the goniometer that will move in relation to the subject's movement during the test. The movement arm is set with the ending position.

RANGE OF MOTION ASSESSMENT OVERVIEW

Prior to beginning the assessment, the client should be provided with a demonstration of a sample ROM test on a joint to explain the assessment process. As each joint's ROM is assessed, the proper starting position, performance of the ROM test, and ending position should all be demonstrated. The following process to position the goniometer occurs before the onset of the assessment:

- Locate the fulcrum at the joint axis or hinge point where the axis of rotation occurs for the two body segments involved.

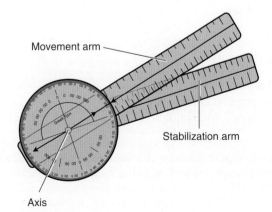

■ **FIGURE 6.5.** A goniometer, including the body axis or fulcrum, a stabilization arm, and a movement arm.

- Place the stabilization and movement arms so that they are centered along each body segment according to the landmarks for each joint measurement (note that the goniometer arms should be long enough to properly align with the landmarks).

The stationary arm of the goniometer will need to be stabilized while the movement arm moves with the body segment through the ROM. The client should be instructed to move the body segment slowly through the ROM until the body segment cannot move further without causing discomfort or shifting other body parts. When there is no further movement, the joint angle is measured and recorded. The use of goniometry can be an accurate measure of a joint's ROM when the following procedures are properly performed (4):

- All anatomic landmarks are identified.
- The joint axis point has been clearly defined.
- The body is stabilized in proper alignment from the start to ending positions.
- The client is instructed to move slowly through the proper ROM, and the goniometer remains aligned to each body segment.
- Measurements are read and recorded correctly.
- The test administrator is familiar with the normal ROM for each joint structure.
- Careful observations are made whether each joint's ROM assessment is pain free.

SPECIFIC RANGE OF MOTION TESTS

In all ROM assessments, locations of the goniometer for the following three points need to be clearly specified to ensure accurate measurements:

1. Fulcrum
2. Stabilization arm
3. Movement arm

Additionally, stabilization of surrounding body parts must occur, and starting and ending body positions must be defined and measured precisely. In the following section are specifications for the various ROM assessments of the shoulder and the hip. An average ROM for each assessment is also provided in *Table 6.3*.

Structure: The Shoulder

Movement: Flexion

Goniometer position (Fig. 6.6)

1. Fulcrum: lateral aspect of greater tubercle
2. Stabilization arm: perpendicular to the floor
3. Movement arm: aligned with midline of humerus and referenced with the lateral epicondyle

Stabilization: Client is in good posture with a stabilized scapula (retracted) and thoracic and lumbar spine. Stabilize scapula to prevent tilting, rotation, or elevation.
Starting/ending body position: Client is seated with glenohumeral in 0 degrees of flexion, extension, abduction, or adduction. Head is in neutral position. Palm of hand should face the body. Elbow should be extended completely. Client performs glenohumeral flexion until the first sign of resistance. (Note: This can also be performed with client starting in supine position, with hips and knees flexed.)

TABLE 6.3. Range of Motion of Select Single Joint Movements in Degrees			
	Degrees		**Degrees**
Shoulder Girdle Movement			
Flexion	90–120	Extension	20–60
Abduction	80–100		
Horizontal abduction	30–45	Horizontal adduction	90–135
Medial rotation	70–90	Lateral rotation	70–90
Elbow Movement			
Flexion	135–160		
Supination	75–90	Pronation	75–90
Trunk Movement			
Flexion	120–150	Extension	20–45
Lateral flexion	10–35	Rotation	20–40
Hip Movement			
Flexion	90–135	Extension	10–30
Abduction	30–50	Adduction	10–30
Medial rotation	30–45	Lateral rotation	45–60
Knee Movement			
Flexion	130–140	Extension	5–10
Ankle Movement			
Dorsiflexion	15–20	Plantarflexion	30–50
Inversion	10–30	Eversion	10–20

Adapted from (7).

Movement: Extension

Goniometer position (Fig. 6.7)

1. Fulcrum: lateral aspect of greater tubercle
2. Stabilization arm: perpendicular to the floor
3. Movement arm: aligned with midline of the lateral humerus and referenced with the lateral epicondyle

   Stabilization: Client is in good posture with a stabilized scapula (retracted) and thoracic and lumbar spine. Stabilize scapula to prevent tilting, rotation, or elevation. Place towel under humerus to stabilize and align with acromion process.
   Starting/ending body position: Client is prone on table with glenohumeral in 0 degrees of flexion, extension, abduction, or adduction. Head is in neutral position. Palm of hand should face the body. Elbow should be extended completely. Client performs glenohumeral extension until the first sign of resistance.

Movement: Internal Rotation

Goniometer position (Fig. 6.8)

1. Fulcrum: olecranon process of the elbow
2. Stabilization arm: perpendicular to the floor

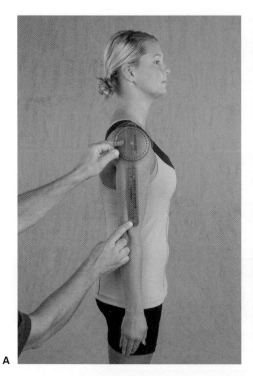

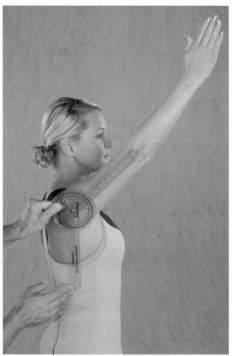

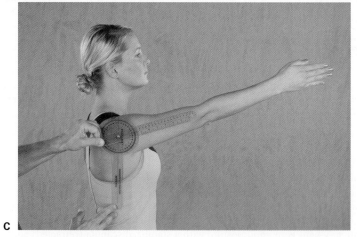

■ **FIGURE 6.6.** Shoulder flexion range of motion.

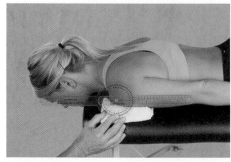

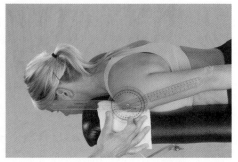

■ **FIGURE 6.7.** Shoulder extension range of motion.

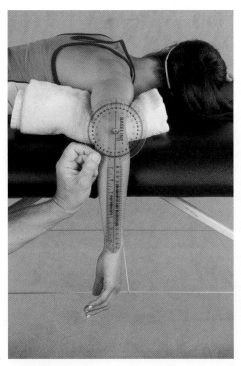
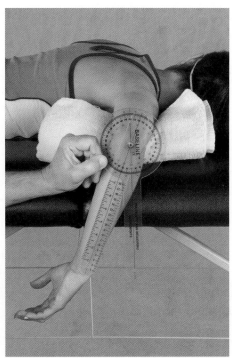

A   B

■ **FIGURE 6.8.** Shoulder rotation — internal range of motion.

3. Movement arm: aligned with lateral midline of ulna and referenced with the ulnar styloid

   Stabilization: Place towel under humerus to stabilize and align with acromion process.
   Starting/ending body position: Client is in prone position with humerus abducted at 90 degrees and elbow flexed at 90 degrees. Client performs internal rotation (moving palm upward) until the first sign of resistance.

Movement: External Rotation

Goniometer position (Fig. 6.9)

1. Fulcrum: olecranon process of the elbow
2. Stabilization arm: perpendicular to the floor
3. Movement arm: aligned with lateral midline of ulna and referenced with the ulnar styloid

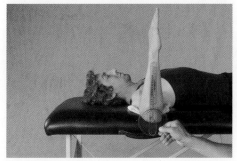
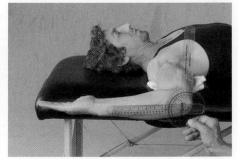

A   B

■ **FIGURE 6.9.** Shoulder rotation — external range of motion.

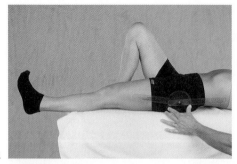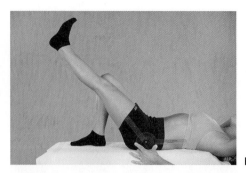

A   B

■ **FIGURE 6.10.** Hip flexion range of motion.

Stabilization: Client is in good posture with a stabilized scapula (retracted) and thoracic and lumbar spine. Place towel under humerus aligned with acromion process to stabilize scapula to prevent tilting, rotation, or elevation.

Starting/ending body position: Client is in supine position with humerus abducted at 90 degrees and elbow flexed at 90 degrees. Client performs external rotation (lowering forearm with palm facing upward) until the first sign of resistance.

Structure: The Hip

Movement: Flexion

Goniometer position (Fig. 6.10)

1. Fulcrum: greater trochanter of the lateral thigh
2. Stabilization arm: lateral midline of the pelvis
3. Movement arm: lateral midline of the femur, using the lateral epicondyle as a reference

Stabilization: Client is in good posture with a stabilized scapula, thoracic and lumbar spine, and pelvic area. Pelvis should not rise off the table. Opposite leg not being assessed should have knee extended on the table for added stability and protection for the back.

Starting/ending body position: Client is supine on the table with hip in 90 degrees of flexion and knee in 90 degrees of flexion (the knee is flexed to reduce contraction of hamstrings). Client performs hip flexion until the first sign of resistance or until the pelvis rotates.

Movement: Extension

Goniometer position (Fig. 6.11)

1. Fulcrum: greater trochanter of the lateral thigh
2. Stabilization arm: lateral midline of the pelvis

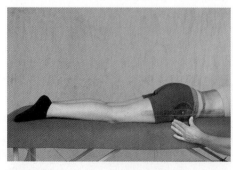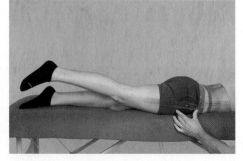

A   B

■ **FIGURE 6.11.** Hip extension range of motion.

3. Movement arm: lateral midline of the femur, using the lateral epicondyle as a reference

Stabilization: Client is in good posture with a stabilized scapula, thoracic and lumbar spine, and pelvic area. Pelvis should not rise off the table. Opposite leg not being assessed should have leg fully extended on the table for added stability.

Starting/ending body position: Client is prone on the table with hip in 0 degrees of flexion, extension, abduction, adduction, and rotation. Testing leg has knee fully extended. Client performs hip extension until the first sign of resistance or until the pelvis rotates.

Movement: Abduction

Goniometer position (Fig. 6.12)

1. Fulcrum: located at the anterior superior iliac spine (ASIS)
2. Stabilization arm: imaginary horizontal line connecting axis point ASIS to the other ASIS
3. Movement arm: anterior midline of the femur, using the midline of the patella as a reference

Stabilization: Client is in good posture with a stabilized scapula, thoracic and lumbar spine, and pelvic area. Stabilize for lateral trunk flexion on both sides.

Starting/ending body position: Client is supine on the table with hip in 0 degrees of flexion, extension, and rotation. Testing leg has knee fully extended. Client performs hip abduction until the first sign of resistance or lateral trunk flexion occurs on either side.

Movement: Adduction

Goniometer position (Fig. 6.13)

1. Fulcrum: located at the ASIS
2. Stabilization arm: imaginary horizontal line connecting axis point ASIS to the other ASIS

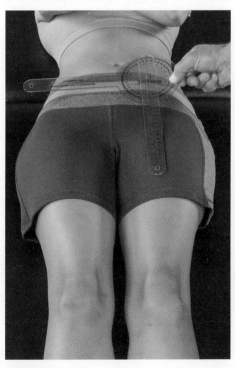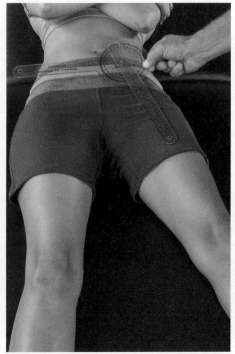

A   B

■ **FIGURE 6.12.** Hip abduction range of motion.

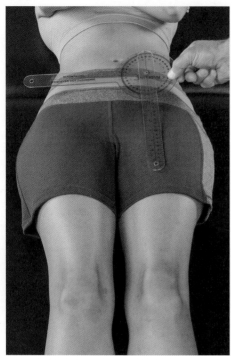 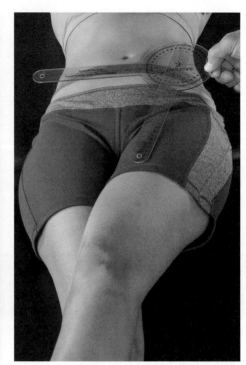

A

B

■ **FIGURE 6.13.** Hip adduction range of motion.

3. Movement arm: anterior midline of the femur, using the midline of the patella as a reference

Stabilization: Client is in good posture with a stabilized scapula, thoracic and lumbar spine, and pelvic area. Opposite leg not being tested should be abducted fully to allow for testing hip to be assessed.

Starting/ending body position: Client is supine on the table with hip in 0 degrees of flexion, extension, and rotation. Testing leg has knee fully extended. Client performs hip adduction until the first sign of resistance or lateral trunk flexion or pelvic rotation occurs.

INTERPRETATION

Reference ranges for ROM measurements are shown in *Table 6.3*. There are no universally accepted standards for ROM and thus it is quite possible that some facilities or programs may use alternate reference ranges.

It is important to recognize that a learning effect is likely with flexibility measurements.

A recommendation from the American Medical Association (1) suggests that ROM should be measured using three consecutive trials and averaged as the true value. If the average ROM is <50 degrees, three of the measurements must fall within ±5 degrees of the mean. If the average is ≥50 degrees, three measurements must fall within ±10 degrees of average. Such measures may be taken up to six times until they meet the criteria; otherwise, they are considered invalid.

SUMMARY

Similar to the HRPF assessment of muscular endurance, there is no one single measurement that provides an overall measurement of flexibility. Fortunately, goniometer assessments are quite feasible, which provides a great opportunity to perform these assessments with clients. Fitness professionals are increasingly incorporating flexibility assessments in their evaluation of clients' HRPF.

LABORATORY ACTIVITIES

RANGE OF MOTION ASSESSMENTS

Data Collection

Work with one other student (he or she measures you, you measure him or her) to perform the following ROM assessments. The measure is taken passively as the movement is slowly and gradually performed until maximum range is achieved as evidenced by high mechanical resistance or the discomfort of the subject.

Movement	Right	Left
Hip flexion	_____	_____
Hip extension	_____	_____
Hip adduction	_____	_____
Hip abduction	_____	_____
Shoulder flexion	_____	_____
Shoulder extension	_____	_____
Shoulder internal rotation	_____	_____
Shoulder external rotation	_____	_____

Written Report

Provide an interpretation of your ROM for each measured movement. Highlight any results that were not within the expected average range for each measure. Were there any imbalances between assessments on the right versus the left side of the body? Comment on what problems could arise from poor flexibility test scores from these measurements.

DISTANCE TESTS FOR FLEXIBILITY ASSESSMENT

Data Collection

Work with one other student (he or she measures you, you measure him or her) to perform the following distance tests of flexibility assessments. The measure is taken passively as the movement is slowly and gradually performed until maximum range is achieved as evidenced by high mechanical resistance or the discomfort of the subject.

Sit-and-Reach Test
Trial 1: _____   Trial 2: _____   Trial 3: _____   Best score: _____

Lumbar flexion:
Trial 1: _____   Trial 2: _____   Trial 3: _____   Best score: _____

Lumbar extension:
Trial 1: _____   Trial 2: _____   Trial 3: _____   Best score: _____

Written Report

Provide an interpretation of your flexibility for each test. Comment on what problems could arise from poor flexibility test scores from these measurements.

CASE STUDY

Jill stopped by a booth at a local health fair and had a flexibility assessment. Jill, who is 33 yr of age, scored in the well-above-average category for this sit-and-reach test. Jill was given a copy of the report, which stated that her flexibility was "excellent." As her fitness consultant, Jill brings a copy of this report to you. What should you tell Jill about this report and this health-related physical fitness component?

REFERENCES

1. American Medical Association. *Guides to the Evaluation of Permanent Impairment.* 4th ed. Chicago (IL): American Medical Association; 1993. 339 p.
2. Canadian Society for Exercise Physiology. *The Canadian Physical Activity, Fitness & Lifestyle Approach (CPAFLA): CSEP—Health & Fitness Program's Health-Related Appraisal and Counselling Strategy.* 3rd ed. Ottawa (Ontario): Canadian Society for Exercise Physiology; 2003. 300 p.
3. Clarkson HM. *Musculoskeletal Assessment: Joint Range of Motion and Manual Muscle Strength.* 2nd ed. Philadelphia (PA): Lippincott Williams & Wilkins; 2000. 415 p.
4. Griffin JC. Client-centered musculoskeletal assessments. In: Wilgren S, Mustain E, Grahm M, editors. *Client-Centered Exercise Prescription.* Champaign: Human Kinetics; 1998. 264 p.
5. Jackson AW, Morrow JR Jr, Brill PA, Kohl HW 3rd, Gordon NF, Blair SN. Relations of sit-up and sit-and-reach tests to low back pain in adults. *J Orthop Sports Phys Ther.* 1998;27:22–6.
6. Lea R, Gerhardt J. Current concepts review. Range of motion measurements. *J Bone Joint Surg.* 1995;77(5):784–98.
7. Norkin CC, Levangie PK. *Joint Structure & Function: A Comprehensive Analysis.* 2nd ed. Philadelphia (PA): Davis; 1992. 512 p.
8. YMCA of the USA, Golding LA. *YMCA Fitness Testing and Assessment Manual.* 4th ed. Champaign (IL): Human Kinetics; 2000. 247 p.

Cardiorespiratory Fitness: Estimation from Field and Submaximal Exercise Tests

WHY MEASURE CARDIORESPIRATORY FITNESS?

Cardiorespiratory fitness (CRF) reflects the functional capabilities of the heart, blood vessels, lungs, and skeletal muscles to perform work. As such, it is often considered one of the best indicators of the collective health and function of the entire body. CRF is the ability to perform large-muscle, dynamic, moderate-to-high intensity exercise for prolonged periods. There are many different terms that have been used to describe this measure of physical fitness, including the following:

- Maximal aerobic capacity
- Functional capacity
- Physical work capacity (PWC)
- Cardiovascular endurance, fitness, or capacity
- Cardiorespiratory endurance, fitness, or capacity
- Cardiopulmonary endurance, fitness, or capacity

There are a multitude of desirable outcomes that can be derived from the assessment of CRF. Some of these outcomes are derived from additional measurements (*e.g.*, an electrocardiogram) that are recorded during the exercise test when determining CRF. Purely from a fitness perspective, CRF can be used to provide motivation for an individual considering participation in a physical activity/exercise program, to individualize the exercise prescription, and to track progress within an exercise program.

Another important value of the assessment of CRF is that it directly relates to an individual's functional status, as noted by use of the term functional capacity to describe CRF. This can be demonstrated in part by comparing a 45-yr-old woman with high (85th percentile) CRF fitness (11.4 metabolic equivalents [METs]) to one with low (15th percentile) CRF fitness (7.6 METs). The highly fit woman can easily perform occupational and recreational activities that require 6–9 METS, such as carrying groceries upstairs, riding a bicycle at 10 mph, shoveling snow, or playing singles tennis (1). The woman with low fitness will only be able to perform these same activities, if at all, with maximal or near-maximal effort and will fatigue quickly. Two other functional reasons for assessing CRF involve clinical decisions regarding work. CRF results can aid in making occupational disability determinations and can also provide a component of a return to work evaluation for individuals with an occupation that involves regular aerobic activity. Finally, CRF, in combination with other exercise test measurements, can provide valuable clinical information, both prognostic and diagnostic, for patients with or without chronic diseases. *Chapter 5* of *ACSM's Guidelines for Exercise Testing and Prescription, Ninth Edition (GETP9)* contains an excellent summary of the clinical use of the exercise test. Indeed, this section summarizes the evidence that establishes a low level of CRF as an independent risk factor for all-cause and cardiovascular mortality. *ACSM's GETP9* highlights, among others, the following two research studies, which clearly demonstrate the importance of CRF:

> *Kodama et al. (12) performed a meta-analysis that collectively included 33 studies totaling over 100,000 subjects and 6,000 all-cause mortality and 4,000 cardiovascular events. They found estimated aerobic capacity from treadmill speed and grade or ergometer workload was a consistent prognostic marker in apparently healthy men and women. Each 1 MET increase in aerobic capacity reflected a 13% decrease in all-cause mortality and 15% decrease in cardiovascular events. Myers et al. (18) examined a large cohort of >3,000 men with variable CVD risk factors with and without confirmed disease and found aerobic capacity was a superior predictor of mortality when compared to tobacco use, hypertension, elevated lipids, and diabetes mellitus.*

WHAT IS THE GOLD STANDARD TEST?

The gold standard measure of CRF is the maximal exercise test with collection of expired gases. This test is performed in a laboratory setting, with trained personnel, using specific monitoring equipment. Maximal exercise testing will be covered in *Chapter 8*. Because this method involves time, expense, and skilled personnel as well as a higher level of risk, it is not always feasible or desired. It should be noted that maximal exercise testing is also performed in clinical settings for diagnosis and prognosis of some chronic diseases. Fortunately, there are many alternative approaches to provide estimates of CRF. These alternative assessment tests for CRF fall into two categories:

1. Field tests: These tests can occur in various nonlaboratory settings (*i.e.*, in the "field") and can typically be administered to a group of people simultaneously. Most commonly, these tests require clients to complete a certain distance as quickly as possible, or to cover as much distance as possible in a fixed amount of time, or to perform a set amount of work in a fixed amount of time.
2. Submaximal exercise tests: These exercise tests limit the level of effort to submaximal exertion. These tests are typically performed in a laboratory setting by one client at a time.

DECIDING ON WHICH METHOD TO USE

The fitness professional needs to assist the client in determining which test may be the most appropriate for CRF assessment. Because the alternative tests involve the prediction of CRF, the standard error of estimate (SEE), as discussed in *Chapter 1*, is part of the decision process. Other factors that may influence the test selection decision are the following:

- Time required
- Expense
- Personnel required
- Equipment and facilities required
- Risk level

PRETEST STANDARDIZATIONS FOR CARDIORESPIRATORY FITNESS ASSESSMENTS

To obtain optimal results, pretest instructions for clients to follow prior to performing a CRF assessment test should be provided. Clients should be instructed to wear comfortable exercise-type clothing, avoid tobacco and caffeine 3 h prior to the test, avoid alcohol 12 h prior to the test, consume plenty of fluids and avoid strenuous exercise for 24 h prior to the test, and obtain an adequate amount of sleep the night before the test.

The informed consent process should be completed, and performance instructions specific to the test should be reviewed with the client. It is crucial that the client understands that he or she is free to terminate the test at any time and is also responsible for informing the test administrator of any and all symptoms that might develop. Also, if used, an explanation of the rating of perceived exertion (RPE) scale is warranted at this time. This scale, developed by Gunnar Borg, is provided in *Table 4.7* of *ACSM's GETP9*. Verbal directions should be read to the client prior to the test for obtaining the RPE measurement. These directions should be consistent with the recommendations of Borg (5).

FIELD TESTS FOR PREDICTION OF AEROBIC CAPACITY

Many field tests originated from physical education curricula that desired to assess CRF of a large group of students at the same time in a nonlaboratory, or field, setting. Field tests have several advantages. They do not require highly trained personnel to administer them, they are time efficient (many tested in one session), and they are inexpensive, requiring little, if any, equipment. Generally, these types of tests are considered safe to perform; however, this may be because they are typically used in younger, low-risk populations. It is important to recognize that some of the tests, such as running 1.5 mi as rapidly as possible, will result in a maximal or near-maximal level of exertion. This requirement may be inappropriate for individuals at moderate-to-high risk for cardiovascular or musculoskeletal complications. Performing the screening procedures reviewed in *Chapter 2* on all clients prior to a CRF assessment and following the personnel recommendations for supervision are thus warranted.

STEP TESTS

The original Harvard two-step test was first used in medicine to aid in the diagnosis of heart disease (17). Many alternative methods have been developed; however, most involve a client performing a fixed amount of work in a set amount of time, followed by the measurement of heart rate response. This manual reviews the McArdle or Queens College step test, which has been commonly used to simultaneously test large groups of students to predict their CRF (16). The procedures for the Queens College step test are provided in *Box 7.1*. Note that any changes to the procedure, including using a different step height or a different rate of stepping, will invalidate the results.

BOX 7.1   Queens College Step Test Procedures

1. The step test requires that the individual step up and down on a standardized step height of 16.25 in (41.25 cm) for 3 min. (Many gymnasium bleachers have a riser height of 16.25 in.)

2. Men step at a rate (cadence) of 24 per minute, whereas women step at a rate of 22 per minute. This cadence should be closely monitored and set with the use of an electronic metronome. A 24-step-per-minute cadence means that the complete cycle of step up with one leg, step up with the other, step down with the first leg, and finally step down with the last leg is performed 24 times in a minute. Commonly the metronome is set at a cadence of four times the step rate, in this case 96 bpm for men, to coordinate each leg's movement with a beat of the metronome. The women's step cadence would be 88 bpm. Although it may be possible to test more than one client at a time, the group would need to be of the same gender.

3. At the conclusion of 3 min, the client stops and palpates the pulse (typically at the radial site) while standing within the first 5 s. A 15-s pulse count is then taken and multiplied by four to determine heart rate (HR) in bpm. This recovery HR should occur within the first 30 s of immediate recovery from the end of the step test. The subject's $\dot{V}O_{2max}$ is determined from the recovery HR by the following formulas:

$$\text{For men: } \dot{V}O_{2max} \ (mL \cdot kg^{-1} \cdot min^{-1}) = 111.33 - (0.42 \times HR)$$

$$\text{For women: } \dot{V}O_{2max} \ (mL \cdot kg^{-1} \cdot min^{-1}) = 65.81 - (0.1847 \times HR)$$

$$HR = \text{recovery HR (bpm)}$$

For example, if a man finished the test with a recovery HR = 144 bpm (36 beats in 15 s), then:

$$\dot{V}O_{2max} \ (mL \cdot kg^{-1} \cdot min^{-1}) = 111.33 - (0.42 \times 144)$$
$$= 50.85 \ mL \cdot kg^{-1} \cdot min^{-1}$$

The Queens College step test is also known as the McArdle step test (11).

FIXED DISTANCE TESTS

There are two common field test protocols that predict CRF by using a walk or run performance of a fixed distance. The performance tests can be classified into two groups: walk/run tests or pure walk tests. In the walk/run test, the subject can walk, run, or use a combination of both to complete the test. In the pure walking tests, subjects are strictly limited to walking the entire test.

The 1-mi walk test is generally indicated for those who have been sedentary or irregularly active or are unable to run because of an injury. The client should be able to walk briskly for 1 mi to be a good candidate for this test.

The 1-mi walk test requires that the subject walk 1 mi as quickly as possible around a measured course. Walking is defined as having one foot in contact with the ground at all times (running involves an airborne phase). The test requires an accurate measure of body weight and a clock to time both the duration of the walk and a 15-s pulse count following the walk. A heart rate (HR) monitor is preferred to a pulse count if one is available. Immediately following the 1-mi walk, the time to complete the test and the HR at the end of the test are recorded. If pulse palpation is used, the client counts the recovery pulse for 15 s and multiplies by four to determine a 1-min recovery HR (beats per minute [bpm]). It is important to have the pulse count completed in the first 20–30 s after the end of the 1-mi walk, and the subject should keep the legs moving to prevent pooling of blood in the periphery, which could lead to light-headedness. The formula to calculate estimated CRF is provided in *Box 7.2* (11). A modified

---

BOX 7.2   Prediction of Cardiorespiratory Fitness from the 1-Mi Walk Test

$$\dot{V}O_{2max} \ (mL \cdot kg^{-1} \cdot min^{-1}) = 132.853 - (0.1692 \times wt) - (0.3877 \times age)$$
$$+ \ (6.315 \times gender) - (3.2649 \times time) - (0.1565 \times HR)$$

Wt = weight in kilograms

Age = in years

Gender = 0 (women) or 1 (men)

Time = in minutes (remember to convert seconds to minutes by dividing by 60)
(*e.g.*, [42/60 = 0.7])

HR = recovery heart rate (HR) in bpm

EXAMPLE
A 32-yr-old man who weighed 170 lb completed the test in 12 min and 36 s with a 15-s pulse count of 35 bpm.

Conversions:

Weight pounds to kilograms: 170/2.2 = 77.3 kg

Time to minutes: 12 + (36/60) = 12.6 min

Pulse in 15 s to HR: 35 × 4 = 140 bpm

$$\dot{V}O_{2max} \ (mL \cdot kg^{-1} \cdot min^{-1}) = 132.853 - (0.1692 \times 77.3) - (0.3877 \times 32)$$
$$+ \ (6.315 \times 1) - (3.2649 \times 12.6) - (0.1565$$
$$\times \ 140) = 50.6 \ mL \cdot kg^{-1} \cdot min^{-1}$$

This formula was derived on apparently healthy individuals ranging in age from 30–69 yr of age (11).

version of this test for use in a swimming pool is also available and could be better suited for those who regularly perform aquatic exercise (10).

The 1.5-mi run test requires the client to complete this distance in the shortest time possible either by running the whole distance, if possible, or by combining running with periods of walking. Ideally, the client should be able to jog for 15 min continuously to obtain a reasonable prediction of CRF. This test is best performed on a track and requires only a stopwatch/clock to administer.

It is important prior to either of the timed distance tests to inform the client of the purpose of the test (*i.e.*, to estimate CRF) and to emphasize that it is critical to find the best pace to cover the specific distance in the shortest amount of time possible. Effective pacing and subject motivation are key determinants in the outcome of this test. For many people, especially those who do not exercise regularly, finding the ideal pace takes practice. Thus, because a learning effect is likely for most people, it is ideal to perform these tests more than once to obtain a better estimate of CRF.

An estimate of maximal volume of oxygen consumed per unit time ($\dot{V}O_{2max}$) from the 1.5-mi run test time is derived from the following formula:

$$\dot{V}O_{2max} \ (mL \cdot kg^{-1} \cdot min^{-1}) = 3.5 + 483/1.5 \ mi \ time \ (min)$$

FIXED TIME TESTS

Another variation of the 1.5-mi run test is the 12-min walk/run test popularized by Dr. Ken Cooper of the Cooper Aerobics Clinic in Dallas, Texas. This test requires the client to cover the maximum distance in 12 min by walking, running, or using a combination of both. The distance covered in 12 min needs to be measured and expressed in meters.

The prediction of CRF from the 12-min walk/run test is:

$$\dot{V}O_{2max} \ (mL \cdot kg^{-1} \cdot min^{-1}) = (distance \ in \ meters - 504.9)/44.73$$

A modified version of this test for swimming is also available (6).

In clinical populations who are very deconditioned, another fixed distance test is commonly performed. The 6-min walk test is a common procedure used as an outcome measure to evaluate progress in rehabilitation programs. Although it is considered a good indicator of functional capacity in these patients, it has generally not been a good predictor of measured $\dot{V}O_{2max}$ (13).

SUBMAXIMAL EXERCISE TESTS

A submaximal exercise test is one that requires the client to perform a fixed amount of work per unit of time. In many cases, these tests require multiple stages or levels. The key distinguishing feature of these tests is that they limit the client's effort to less than maximal exertion. There are several protocols that may be used to conduct a laboratory submaximal exercise test for the prediction of CRF using various testing modalities, from the bench step, to the cycle, to the treadmill. Although some versions of step tests are done on individuals in a medical/fitness office setting, this form of administration is much less common than the use of the test within a field setting. Thus, the step test, as used by groups of students, is classified as a field test within this manual.

PREDICTING MAXIMAL HEART RATE

A fundamental feature of many submaximal exercise tests is the reliance on knowing the client's maximal HR value (HR_{max}). The measurement of HR_{max} requires a maximal exercise effort; thus, it cannot be obtained during submaximal exercise tests. Therefore, these submaximal testing procedures depend on the use of a prediction of HR_{max}, typically estimated from age. Although there are many different prediction equations for HR_{max} (see *Table 7.2* of *ACSM's GETP9*), most have SEE ranges of between ±10 and 15 bpm. The most commonly used equation for predicting HR_{max} is:

$$\text{Age-predicted } HR_{max} = 220 - \text{age (yr)}$$

A meta-analysis performed in 2001 by Tanaka et al. (21) included 18,712 subjects. This investigation confirmed the strong inverse relationship between age and HR_{max}, reporting an r value of −0.90 and provided the following equation:

$$\text{Age-predicted } HR_{max} = 208 - 0.7 \text{ (age)}$$

These prediction equations do work well for groups. For example, if the HR_{max} of 100 40-yr-olds were measured, the average HR_{max} for the group would be very close to 180 bpm. However, approximately one in three people in this group will have a true HR_{max} of either <165 bpm or >195 bpm. This large variability in age-predicted HR_{max} is one of the sources of error in predicting CRF from submaximal exercise tests. Some actual measured HR_{max} at different ages are shown in *Figure 7.1* (23).

TEST TERMINATION CRITERIA

Prior to the onset of the test, clear exercise test endpoints should be established. One recommendation is to use a test termination criterion of 85% of age-predicted HR_{max}. This method should result in a submaximal effort for most clients. However, it needs to be understood that other clients with actual HR_{max} below (2 SEE) the age-predicted average will reach their actual HR_{max}. Thus, observing other signs and symptoms of maximal effort may warrant termination of the test prior to attaining

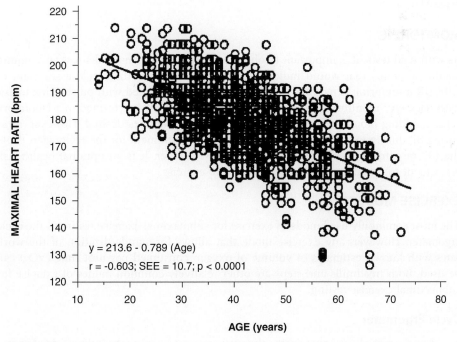

■ FIGURE 7.1. Variability in maximal heart rate at different ages. SEE, standard error of estimate. (Reprinted from [23].)

BOX 7.3   General Indications for Stopping an Exercise Test[a]

- Onset of angina or angina-like symptoms
- Drop in SBP of ≥10 mm Hg with an increase in work rate or if SBP decreases below the value obtained in the same position prior to testing
- Excessive rise in BP: systolic pressure >250 mm Hg and/or diastolic pressure >115 mm Hg
- Shortness of breath, wheezing, leg cramps, or claudication
- Signs of poor perfusion: light-headedness, confusion, ataxia, pallor, cyanosis, nausea, or cold and clammy skin
- Failure of HR to increase with increased exercise intensity
- Noticeable change in heart rhythm by palpation or auscultation
- Subject requests to stop
- Physical or verbal manifestations of severe fatigue
- Failure of the testing equipment

[a]Assumes that testing is nondiagnostic and is being performed without direct physician involvement or ECG monitoring. For clinical testing, *Box 8.1* provides more definitive and specific termination criteria.
BP, blood pressure; ECG, electrocardiogram; HR, heart rate; SBP, systolic blood pressure.

---

the test termination criteria of 85% of age-predicted HR$_{max}$. Additionally, the American College of Sports Medicine (ACSM) has developed a list of indications for stopping an exercise test in adults determined to be in the low-risk stratification category, as noted in *Box 7.3*. As noted at the bottom of *Box 7.3*, there are other test termination criteria used in clinical exercise testing. These criteria will be discussed in *Chapter 8* but may need to be applied in submaximal testing if the client is in the moderate- or high-risk classification.

MONITORING

As with field tests, it is important to observe the client for signs of distress and inquire about symptoms that would indicate test termination. For the actual assessment of CRF, HR monitoring is required, and this can be accomplished with pulse palpation or with telemetry monitoring. Because these tests are typically performed in a laboratory setting, adding blood pressure (BP) monitoring is sometimes desired. However, measuring BP during exercise involves a higher skill requirement for the technician. Note that BP monitoring is not used to estimate CRF; rather, it is an optional health risk assessment to evaluate a client's BP response to exercise.

EXERCISE MODES

The most commonly used mode of exercise for submaximal exercise testing is the cycle ergometer. However, any exercise mode that allows for standardization of the work rates with known estimates of volume of oxygen consumed per unit time ($\dot{V}O_2$) can be used. Both treadmills and steps are other relatively common modes of exercise for submaximal exercise testing.

Cycle Ergometer

There are several advantages to using the cycle ergometer that make it the mode of choice for submaximal exercise testing. One advantage to the cycle is the non–weight-bearing mode of exercise provided, making it a good choice for individuals with orthopedic limitations. Also, the cycle ergometer is a relatively safe mode of exercise because there is less danger of falling off the apparatus as compared to a treadmill or even a step. BP and pulse by palpation are easily measured during exercise on the cycle ergometer because of the limited noise that the cycle produces as well as the natural stabilization of the upper body and arm. Additionally, cycle ergometers are less expensive and more portable than treadmills, require little space, and most have no electrical needs.

There are a few disadvantages with the use of the cycle ergometer that merit consideration. One disadvantage is that a cycle is not a common mode of exercise or activity for many adults in the United States, especially in older populations. Another potential disadvantage is that mechanically braked cycle ergometers require the client to maintain a constant pedaling cadence to keep the work rate constant.

Currently, the mechanically braked Monark cycle ergometer is the most popular brand used for submaximal exercise testing because of the ease in calibrating the ergometer. An example of a mechanically braked cycle ergometer is shown in *Figure* 7.2. Calibration of this ergometer ensures accurate work outputs for the different stages of a submaximal test. The calibration procedure for the Monark cycle ergometer is provided in *Box 7.4*.

Proper seat height is important for optimal performance when using cycle ergometers. The knee should be flexed at approximately 5–10 degrees in the pedal-down position with the client seated with toes on the pedals. *Figure* 7.3 illustrates an incorrect seat height setting, which can result in inefficiency and early fatigue. Another way to check seat height is to have the client first place the heels on the pedals. With the heels on the pedals, the leg should be straight in the pedal-down position. Also, the seat height can be aligned with the client's greater trochanter, or hip, with the client standing next to the cycle. Most importantly, the client should actually sit on the bike, turn the pedals, and evaluate comfort with the seat height. While pedaling, the client should feel comfortable, and there should be no rocking of the hips. Also, the client should maintain an upright posture, which may require an adjustment to the handlebars, and should not grip the handlebars too tightly.

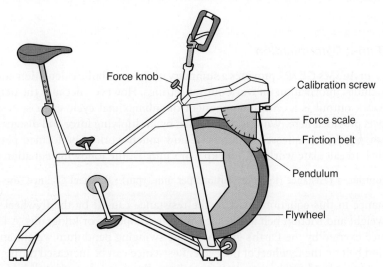

■ **FIGURE 7.2.** The features of a mechanically braked cycle ergometer. (Reprinted from Adams, G. *Exercise Physiology Laboratory Manual*. 3rd ed. New York [NY]: McGraw Hill; 1998. 140 p.)

BOX 7.4	Calibration of the Monark Cycle Ergometer

Prior to calibrating, examine the resistance belt and flywheel for excessive wear and dirt. The flywheel can be cleaned with steel wool and cleanser, and the belt can also be cleaned with a mild detergent. However, you should not conduct a test if either is wet, so plan ahead. Most resistance belts have a lifespan of several years before they need replacing, depending on usage.

The ergometer needs to be on a level surface for the calibration procedure.

1. Loosen or unfasten the resistance belt from the pendulum so that the pendulum hangs free. The line in the center of the pendulum should be in exact alignment with the zero line on the measurement scale. If not, loosen the lock nut to allow movement of the measurement scale to the correct zero point, and then tighten the lock screw to hold this position.
2. Using certified calibration weights (between 3 and 7 kg), hang a known weight to the balancing spring (shorter belt) and check the reading on the measurement scale. If it is not reading the exact weight, adjust the pendulum to the correct weight on the scale by means of the adjusting weight inside the pendulum.
   To change the position of the adjusting weight, loosen the lock screw of the weight. Should the index of the pendulum weight be too low, move the adjusting weight upward in the weight, and if the index should be too high, the adjusting weight is moved somewhat downward and locked in the new position. Repeat until the correct reading is achieved.

When the calibration is completed, reattach the belt to the mechanism and be sure to pull the belt somewhat tightly without too much slack. Check the Monark ergometer handbook[a] for more detailed information about the calibration procedures.

....

[a]Found at http://www.monarkexercise.se/wk_custom/documents/{0f924617-7c92-4710-a13d-6ada7f88f35b}_828_e_manual_en_naetversion_1010.pdf

Work Output Determination

Chapter 7 in *ACSM's GETP9* provides a summary of the metabolic calculation equations, which includes information on work output settings. However, because the determination of work output is a critical component of submaximal cycle exercise testing, an overview is provided here. Work is determined by multiplying force and distance. Work output, or power, is expressed in terms of how much work is performed per unit of time. Thus, to calculate work output ($kp \cdot m \cdot min^{-1}$), the following equation is used:

Work output = resistance (kp) $\cdot$ revolutions per min (rpm) $\cdot$ flywheel distance ($m \cdot rev^{-1}$)

Resistance in this equation refers to the resistance caused by the flywheel by pendulum weight and friction belt and is measured in kiloponds or kilograms. A kilopond is the force exerted by the Earth's gravity by the swinging pendulum weight applied to the friction belt on the flywheel of the cycle. Resistance can be increased during the test to apply standardized work outputs to the client. Because kilopond and kilogram are somewhat interchangeable, the measure of work on the cycle ergometer is commonly expressed as $kg \cdot m \cdot min^{-1}$.

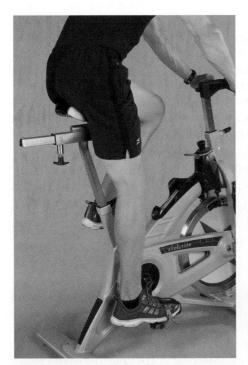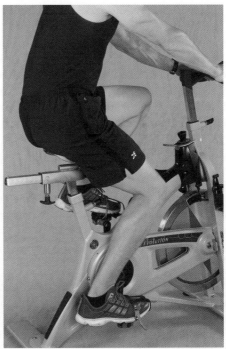

■ **FIGURE 7.3.** An example of a seat height set correctly (left) and too too low (right) for cycle ergometry testing.

Cadence is simply the number of pedal revolutions per minute (rpm). Most common submaximal cycle protocols require a constant rate of 50 rpm. Newer ergometers usually have an electronic console that measures rpm; otherwise, the pedaling rate needs to be in cadence with a metronome set at 100 bpm (100 bpm for 100 downstrokes to produce 50 rpm). It is prudent to periodically verify that the console measure is reading accurately by cross-checking it with a metronome as shown in *Figure 7.4.*

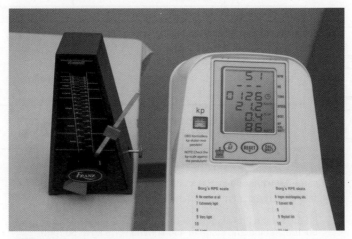

■ **FIGURE 7.4.** The use of a metronome to check the calibration of the revolutions per minute (rpm) meter on a cycle. (Photograph by Ball State University.)

Flywheel travel distance (meters per revolution) is a constant for each type of cycle. The Monark cycle ergometer has a 6 m · rev^{-1} ratio. This means that the flywheel on the Monark cycle will travel 6 m per complete revolution of the pedal (the flywheel is 1.62 m in circumference and travels 3.7 circuits per pedal revolution). If another brand of cycle is used, the flywheel travel distance will need to be verified.

Because the rate is standardized to 50 rpm on the Monark cycle, the client will always be covering 300 m · min^{-1} (50 rpm · 6 m · rev^{-1}). Some examples of some common cycle ergometer work output calculations using the Monark cycle at 50 rpm are as follows:

Resistance setting of 1 kg: 300 kg · m · min^{-1} = 1 kp · 50 rpm · 6 m · rev^{-1}
Resistance setting of 1.5 kg: 450 kg · m · min^{-1} = 1.5 kp · 50 rpm · 6 m · rev^{-1}
Resistance setting of 2 kg: 600 kg · m · min^{-1} = 2 kp · 50 rpm · 6 m · rev^{-1}

It is also important to understand another unit called watts, used to express work output. Watts can be determined from kg · m · min^{-1} by dividing by 6.12 (usually rounded to 6). For example, 600 kg · m · min^{-1} is approximately equal to 100 W.

YMCA SUBMAXIMAL CYCLE TEST

The protocol for the YMCA submaximal cycle test involves a branching, multistage format to gather information to establish a relationship between HR and work rate to ultimately estimate CRF (8). The test requires at least two and possibly four exercise stages (each of 3-min duration), resulting in a total test time between 6 and 12 min. The requirements for the test are to complete two separate workloads that result in HR values between 110 and 150 bpm. As shown in *Figure 7.5*, all subjects start with a first stage workload of 150 kg · m · min^{-1}. The second stage work rate is dependent on the HR value from the first stage.

The recommended procedures for this test are provided in *Box 7.5*. It is important to ensure that the client maintains a pedal rate of 50 ($\pm$2) rpm throughout the test. At each 3-min work stage, a steady-state HR is required, which is operationally defined as an HR at the end of the second and third minute of each stage that does not increase more than

	1st stage	150 kgm/min (0.5 kg)		
	HR: <80	HR: 80–89	HR: 90–100	HR: >100
2nd stage	750 kgm/min (2.5 kg)*	600 kgm/min (2.0 kg)	450 kgm/min (1.5 kg)	300 kgm/min (1.0 kg)
3rd stage	900 kgm/min (3.0 kg)	750 kgm/min (2.5 kg)	600 kgm/min (2.0 kg)	450 kgm/min (1.5 kg)
4th stage	1050 kgm/min (3.5 kg)	900 kgm/min (3.0 kg)	750 kgm/min (2.5 kg)	600 kgm/min (2.0 kg)

Directions:
1 Set the 1st work rate at 150 kgm/min (0.5 kg at 50 rpm)
2 If the HR in the third minute of the stage is:
   <80, set the 2nd stage at 750 kgm/min (2.5 kg at 50 rpm)
   80-89, set the 2nd stage at 600 kgm/min (2.0 kg at 50 rpm)
   90-100, set the 2nd stage at 450 kgm/min (1.5 kg at 50 rpm)
   >100, set the 2nd stage at 300 kgm/min (1.0 kg at 50 rpm)
3 Set the 3rd and 4th (if required) according to the work rates in the columns below the 2nd loads

■ **FIGURE 7.5.** YMCA cycle ergometry protocol.

BOX 7.5	General Procedures for Submaximal Testing of Cardiorespiratory Fitness

1. Obtain resting HR and BP immediately prior to exercise in the exercise posture.
2. The client should be familiarized with the ergometer. If using a cycle ergometer, properly position the client on the ergometer (*i.e.*, upright posture, ~25-degree bend in the knee at maximal leg extension, and hands in proper position on handlebars) (14–16).
3. The exercise test should begin with a 2–3 min warm-up to acquaint the client with the cycle ergometer and prepare him or her for the exercise intensity in the first stage of the test.
4. A specific protocol should consist of 2- or 3-min stages with appropriate increments in work rate.
5. HR should be monitored at least two times during each stage, near the end of the second and third minutes of each stage. If HR is >110 beats · min^{-1}, steady state HR (*i.e.*, two HRs within 5 beats · min^{-1}) should be reached before the workload is increased.
6. BP should be monitored in the last minute of each stage and repeated (verified) in the event of a hypotensive or hypertensive response.
7. RPE (using either the Borg category or category-ratio scale [see *Table 4.7* from *GETP9*]) and additional rating scales should be monitored near the end of the last minute of each stage.
8. Client's appearance and symptoms should be monitored and recorded regularly.
9. The test should be terminated when the subject reaches 70% heart rate reserve (85% of age-predicted HR$_{max}$), fails to conform to the exercise test protocol, experiences adverse signs or symptoms, requests to stop, or experiences an emergency situation.
10. An appropriate cool-down/recovery period should be initiated consisting of either
    a. continued exercise at a work rate equivalent to that of the first stage of the exercise test protocol or lower or
    b. a passive cool-down if the subject experiences signs of discomfort or an emergency situation occurs.
11. All physiologic observations (*e.g.*, HR, BP, signs and symptoms) should be continued for at least 5 min of recovery unless abnormal responses occur, which would warrant a longer posttest surveillance period. Continue low-level exercise until HR and BP stabilize, but not necessarily until they reach preexercise levels.

BP, blood pressure; HR, heart rate; HR$_{max}$, maximal heart rate; RPE, rating of perceived exertion.

5 bpm. If the HR has increased more than 5 bpm, this indicates that the client has not reached steady state, and the stage should be continued for another minute. The resistance setting of the cycle ergometer (provided by the measurement scale on the side of the ergometer) and the pedal rate (50 rpm) should be checked regularly throughout the test and corrected if necessary. Although exercise BP measurements are not required for the computation of CRF, it is suggested that they be taken and recorded at each stage. These data would be used to end a test early in the event a client has a hypertensive or hypotensive response. Further, if the client does in fact have a significantly elevated BP during the test, these data could be valuable for the client's health care professional because an exaggerated BP response to exercise is considered a risk factor for future hypertension (2).

Estimating $\dot{V}O_{2max}$

There are two methods that can be used to derive an estimate of CRF. One involves plotting the data on a graph and using an extrapolation technique, and the other uses a calculation-based formula.

Graphing Technique

The graphing method requires that the two HR and work output data points be plotted on a graph like the one provided in *Figure 7.6*. A horizontal line is drawn across the graph to intersect the y-axis (HR) at the value of age-predicted HR_{max}. Then a straight line connecting the two data points is drawn. This line is extended (extrapolated) up to the horizontal line. Finally, a perpendicular line is drawn down from this point of intersection to the x-axis (work rate). This work rate value is the predicted maximal work rate and is used in the ACSM metabolic equation for leg cycling to calculate a predicted $\dot{V}O_{2max}$.

$$\dot{V}O_2 \ (mL \cdot kg^{-1} \cdot min^{-1}) = [(1.8 \times \text{work rate})/\text{body weight in kilogram}] + 7$$

Figure 7.7 demonstrates the process of graphing the HR response for prediction of $\dot{V}O_{2max}$. This figure also contains an example of how the inaccuracy of age-predicted HR_{max} might influence the results.

Calculation-Based Formula

To calculate a predicted $\dot{V}O_{2max}$, it is necessary to first calculate the slope of the HR and $\dot{V}O_2$ relationship. The slope (a) will then be used within a standard linear regression equation of the form $y = ax + b$, where the y variable represents $\dot{V}O_2$ and where the x variable represents HR.

Calculation of slope:

$$\text{Slope (a)} = (\dot{V}O_2 2 - \dot{V}O_2 1)/(HR2 - HR1)$$

Where

$$\dot{V}O_2 1 = \text{Submaximal predicted } \dot{V}O_2 \text{ from stage 1, in mL} \cdot kg^{-1} \cdot min^{-1}$$
$$\dot{V}O_2 2 = \text{Submaximal predicted } \dot{V}O_2 \text{ from stage 2, in mL} \cdot kg^{-1} \cdot min^{-1}$$
$$HR1 = \text{HR from stage 1, in bpm}$$
$$HR2 = \text{HR from stage 2, in bpm}$$

$\dot{V}O_{2max}$ is then estimated from the following equation:

$$\dot{V}O_{2max}(mL \cdot kg^{-1} \cdot min^{-1}) = a \ (HR_{max} - HR2) + \dot{V}O_2 2$$

Where

$$HR_{max} = 220 - \text{age}$$

For example, a 30-yr-old male (75 kg) completed two stages (450 and 600 kg · m · min^{-1}) with HR values of 116 and 130 bpm, respectively. His $\dot{V}O_{2max}$ would be calculated as follows:

$$\dot{V}O_2 1 \ (mL \cdot kg^{-1} \cdot min^{-1}) = [(1.8 \times \text{work rate})/\text{body weight in kilogram}] + 7$$
$$= [(1.8 \times 450)/75] + 7 = 17.8$$
$$\dot{V}O_2 2 \ (mL \cdot kg^{-1} \cdot min^{-1}) = [(1.8 \times \text{work rate})/\text{body weight in kilogram}] + 7$$
$$= [(1.8 \times 600)/75] + 7 = 21.4$$
$$a = (21.4 - 17.8)(130 - 116) = 0.257$$
$$\dot{V}O_{2max} \ (mL \cdot kg^{-1} \cdot min^{-1}) = a \ (HR_{max} - HR2) + \dot{V}O_2 2$$
$$= [0.257 \ ((220 - 30) - 130)] + 21.4$$
$$= 36.8 \ mL \cdot kg^{-1} \cdot min^{-1}$$

Name: _____   Age: _____   Weight: _____   Predicted Max HR _____

	Date	1st Workload HR >110	2nd Workload HR >110	(Est) Max Workload	(Est) Max O$_2$ (L · min^{-1})	(Est) Max O$_2$ (mL^{-1} · kg^{-1} · min^{-1})
Test #1	_____	_____	_____	_____	_____	_____
Test #2	_____	_____	_____	_____	_____	_____
Test #3	_____	_____	_____	_____	_____	_____

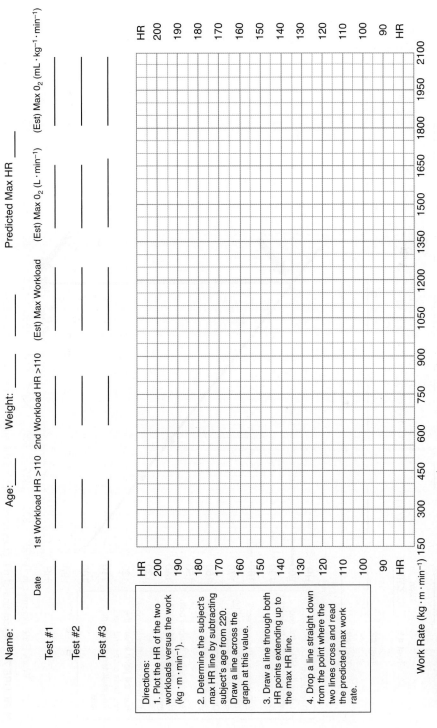

Directions:
1. Plot the HR of the two workloads versus the work (kg · m · min^{-1}).

2. Determine the subject's max HR line by subtracting subject's age from 220. Draw a line across the graph at this value.

3. Draw a line through both HR points extending up to the max HR line.

4. Drop a line straight down from the point where the two lines cross and read the predicted max work rate.

Work Rate (kg · m · min^{-1})

FIGURE 7.6. A graph used for the prediction of $\dot{V}O_{2max}$ from cycle ergometry tests.

Name: ___Pedro___   Age: __20__   Weight: __175 lbs__   Predicted Max HR __200 bpm__

Test #1 Date 10/22/04   1st Workload HR >110 127 bpm   2nd Workload HR >110 141 bpm   (Est) Max Workload 1200 kg · m · min⁻¹   (Est) Max O₂ (L · min⁻¹) _____   (Est) Max O₂ (mL · kg⁻¹ · min⁻¹) 34.2 mL · kg⁻¹ · min⁻¹

Test #2 _____ _____ _____ _____ _____ _____

Test #3 _____ _____ _____ _____ _____ _____

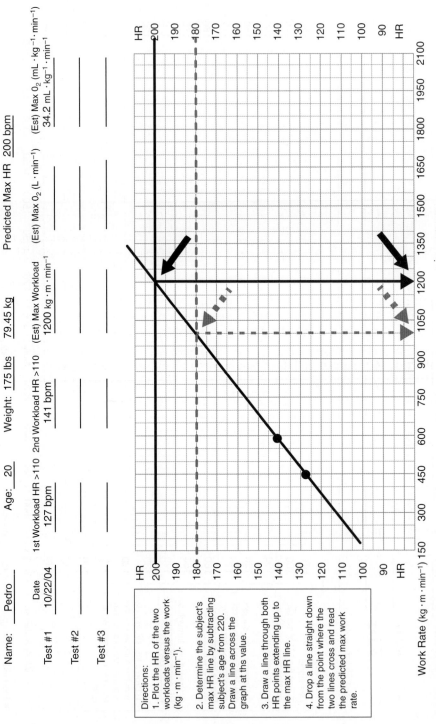

Directions:
1. Plot the HR of the two workloads versus the work (kg · m · min⁻¹).

2. Determine the subject's max HR line by subtracting subject's age from 220. Draw a line across the graph at this value.

3. Draw a line through both HR points extending up to the max HR line.

4. Drop a line straight down from the point where the two lines cross and read the predicted max work rate.

■ **FIGURE 7.7.** Description of the process of graphing the heart rate response for prediction of $\dot{V}O_{2max}$.

TABLE 7.1. Åstrand Cycle Submaximal Cycle Ergometer Test Initial Workloads	
Individual	Work Output (kp · m⁻¹ · min⁻¹)
Men	
Unconditioned	300–600
Conditioned	600–900
Women	
Unconditioned	300–450
Conditioned	450–600
Poorly conditioned or older individuals	300

This protocol table is designed as a guide. The protocol is designed to elicit an HR of between 125 and 170 bpm by 6 min. You can adjust the work output as necessary during the test (usually after the first 6 min) to achieve an HR in or near this range in your subject.

ÅSTRAND SUBMAXIMAL CYCLE ERGOMETER TEST

Per Olaf Åstrand (a noted Swedish exercise physiologist), along with his wife, Irma Ryhming, developed a simple protocol in the 1950s to predict CRF from laboratory submaximal cycle exercise results. This protocol is sometimes known as the Åstrand-Ryhming protocol. The client typically performs one 6-min submaximal exercise stage of a standardized work rate. The work rate is selected according to recommendations found in *Table 7.1*. This procedure requires an exercise HR value between 125 and 170 bpm. Most of the procedures are similar to the YMCA protocol including maintaining a 50 rpm pedal rate and monitoring the client throughout the test. A steady-state HR is required at the end of the 6-min work stage. If the HR is below 125 bpm, then workload is increased, and the test continues for an additional 6 min, making the total test time range the same as for the YMCA protocol.

Estimating $\dot{V}O_{2max}$

There are two methods that can be used to derive an estimate of CRF. One involves plotting the data on a graph called a nomogram, and the other uses a calculation-based formula.

Nomogram Technique

A nomogram is a graphic representation where two known data points are plotted and connected with a line to predict a third, unknown value. *Figure 7.8* depicts a nomogram used for calculating the unknown $\dot{V}O_{2max}$ from the HR during submaximal work (3). Using this nomogram technique, a mark is placed on the HR scale (left side of nomogram) at the steady-state HR (value must be between 125 and 170 bpm). Note that this scale actually has two sides, one for men (left) and one for women (right). Next, a mark is placed on the workload scale (right side of nomogram). Note that this scale also has two sides, one for men (right) and one for women (left). The two points are connected with a straight line, and the $\dot{V}O_{2max}$ is read from the center scale. The correction factor table found in *Table 7.2* must then be used to adjust the $\dot{V}O_{2max}$ for the person's age (nearest 5 yr). For example, if the $\dot{V}O_{2max}$ was estimated to be 3.65 L · min⁻¹ from the nomogram, the corrected value for a 40-yr-old man would be 3.03 L · min⁻¹ (3.65 × 0.83).

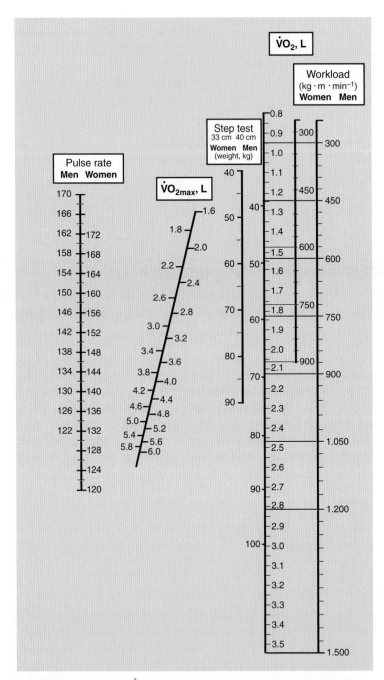

■ FIGURE 7.8. Modified Åstrand-Ryhming nomogram. (From Astrand P-O, Ryhming I. A nomogram for calculation of aerobic capacity [physical fitness] from pulse rate during submaximal work. *J Appl Physiol.* 1954;7:218–21, with permission.)

TABLE 7.2. Age Correction Factor for Åstrand Cycle Ergometer Test Results	
Age	**Correction Factor**
15	1.10
25	1.00
35	0.87
40	0.83
45	0.78
50	0.75
55	0.71
60	0.68
65	0.65

Adapted from American College of Sports Medicine. *ACSM's Health-Related Physical Fitness Assessment Manual.* 2nd ed. Philadelphia (PA): Wolters Kluwer Health Ltd; 2005. 121 p.

Calculation-Based Formula

To calculate the $\dot{V}O_{2max}$ (mL · kg^{-1} · min^{-1}) from the single-stage Åstrand protocol, the following formula is used:

$$\dot{V}O_{2max} \text{ (mL · kg}^{-1} \text{ · min}^{-1}) = \dot{V}O_2 1 \, [(220 - \text{age} - 73 - (G \times 10))/(HR - 73 - (G \times 10))]$$

Where

$$\dot{V}O_2 1 \text{ (submaximal workload)} = [(1.8 \times \text{work rate})/\text{body weight in kilogram}] + 7$$
$$G = 0 \text{ for women and 1 for men}$$
$$HR = \text{steady-state HR, in bpm}$$

For example, calculate $\dot{V}O_{2max}$ for a 33-yr-old conditioned woman (63 kg), with a single stage of 600 kg · m · min^{-1} where the HR value was 124 bpm, as follows:
Solve for $\dot{V}O_2 1$:

$$\dot{V}O_2 1 \text{ (mL · kg}^{-1} \text{ · min}^{-1}) = [(1.8 \times \text{work rate})/\text{body weight in kilogram}] + 7$$
$$= [(1.8 \times 600)/63] + 7 = 24.1$$

Then, insert $\dot{V}O_2 1$ and appropriate gender, age, and HR values into formula:

$$\dot{V}O_{2max} \text{ (mL · kg}^{-1} \text{ · min}^{-1}) = \dot{V}O_2 1 \, [(220 - \text{age} - 73 - (G \times 10))/(HR - 73 - (G \times 10))]$$
$$= 24.1 \, [(220 - 33 - 73 - (0 \times 10))/(124 - 73 - (0 \times 10))]$$
$$= 53.8 \text{ mL · kg}^{-1} \text{ · min}^{-1}$$

TREADMILL

A submaximal treadmill exercise test can also be used to predict CRF. Thus, the same basic principle as used for the YMCA cycle test, namely determining the specific linear relationship between HR and $\dot{V}O_2$, is used to derive the estimate. The same HR range of two work stages with HR values between 110 and 150 bpm is recommended.

Although there are many different treadmill protocols, as will be discussed in *Chapter 8*, a common one used for submaximal assessments is the Bruce protocol. Most clients should be able to obtain two HR values between 110 and 150 bpm within the first three stages (each 3 min in duration) of this protocol. (Note: The entire protocol is found in *Chapter 8, Table 8.3*.)

The basic procedures are identical to the YMCA submaximal cycle protocol with the exception of the mode of exercise. The warm-up minute is performed at 1.7 mph with no elevation. If the client's HR is ≥ 110 bpm at the first stage, then only one additional stage is required. Thus, this test will last between 6 and 9 min.

Estimating $\dot{V}O_{2max}$

$\dot{V}O_{2max}$ is then estimated from the same equation that was used with the YMCA cycle protocol.

$$\dot{V}O_{2max} \text{ (in mL} \cdot \text{kg}^{-1} \cdot \text{min}^{-1}) = a \text{ (HR}_{max} - \text{HR2)} + \dot{V}O_2 2$$

However, the work rate value is now derived from speed (S) and grade (G) on the treadmill and is used in the ACSM metabolic equation to calculate a predicted $\dot{V}O_2$.

$$\dot{V}O_2 \text{ (mL} \cdot \text{kg}^{-1} \cdot \text{min}^{-1}) = [(0.1 \times S) + (1.8 \times S \times G)] + 3.5$$

Where

$$S \text{ (speed)} = \text{mph} \times 26.8 \text{ m} \cdot \text{min}^{-1} \cdot \text{mph}^{-1}$$
$$G \text{ (grade)} = \% \text{ elevation}/100$$

For example, the first stage with a speed of 1.7 mph and a grade of 10% would have a predicted $\dot{V}O_2$ for this stage calculated as follows:

$$\dot{V}O_2 \text{ (mL} \cdot \text{kg}^{-1} \cdot \text{min}^{-1}) = [(0.1 \times [1.7 \times 26.8]) + (1.8 \times [1.7 \times 26.8] \times [10/100])] + 3.5$$
$$= 16.2 \text{ mL} \cdot \text{kg}^{-1} \cdot \text{min}^{-1}$$

INTERPRETATION

Table 7.3 provides normative values for estimated $\dot{V}O_{2max}$ from the YMCA submaximal cycle ergometer test with specific reference to age and sex (8). As indicated earlier in this chapter, the gold standard test for CRF is a maximal exercise test with $\dot{V}O_{2max}$ measured from the collection of expired gases. Because both field tests and submaximal exercise tests require prediction of $\dot{V}O_{2max}$, the interpretation of the results needs to include an expression of SEE. Unfortunately, some of the prediction equations used do not provide an SEE.

SOURCES OF ERROR IN SUBMAXIMAL PREDICTION

There are several potential sources of error in submaximal exercise tests when predicting $\dot{V}O_{2max}$ (4,15). Certainly, any errors in the measurement of workload (this would include using an ergometer that was not properly calibrated) or in the measurement of HR will result in prediction error.

One primary source of error is that associated with age-predicted HR$_{max}$. This variability between individuals was covered earlier, and an example of the potential for error can be observed using *Figure* 7.7 by observing the difference in predicted maximal work rate if the actual HR$_{max}$ was 180 bpm.

A second source of error is the variability in mechanical efficiency on an ergometer. In other words, some people will be more efficient (meaning they will require less O_2 to perform a given work rate). The *ACSM's GETP, Seventh Edition* noted, "The intersubject variability in measured $\dot{V}O_2$ may have a standard error of estimate as high as 7% for performing a given work rate" (22). This value is consistent with the $\pm 6\%$ suggested by Astrand and Rodahl (4).

A third source of error is the variability in submaximal HR at the same work rate on different days. One study by Davies (7) reported that at intensities producing HR between 120 and 150 bpm, the HR varied by $\pm 8\%$ on different days. This is notable

TABLE 7.3. Fitness Categories for Estimated $\dot{V}O_{2max}$ from the YMCA Submaximal Cycle Ergometer Test by Age and Sex

% Ranking		Norms for Max $\dot{V}O_2$ (mL/kg) — MEN					
		Age (year)					
% Ranking		18–25	26–35	36–45	46–55	56–65	Over 65
100		100	95	90	83	65	53
95	Excellent	75	66	61	55	50	42
90		65	60	55	49	43	38
85		60	55	49	45	40	34
80	Good	56	52	47	43	38	33
75		53	50	45	40	37	32
70		50	48	43	39	35	31
65	Above average	49	45	41	38	34	30
60		48	44	40	36	33	29
55		45	42	38	35	32	28
50	Average	44	40	37	33	31	27
45		43	39	36	32	30	26
40		42	38	35	31	28	25
35	Below average	39	37	33	30	27	24
30		38	34	31	29	26	23
25		36	33	30	27	25	22
20	Poor	35	32	29	26	23	21
15		32	30	27	25	22	20
10		30	27	24	24	21	18
5	Very poor	26	24	21	20	18	16
0		20	15	14	13	12	10
% Ranking		Norms for Max $\dot{V}O_2$ (mL/kg) — WOMEN					
		Age (year)					
% Ranking		18–25	26–35	36–45	46–55	56–65	Over 65
100		95	95	75	72	58	55
95	Excellent	69	65	56	51	44	48
90		59	58	50	45	40	34
85		56	53	46	41	36	31
80	Good	52	51	44	39	35	30
75		50	48	42	36	33	29
70		47	45	41	35	32	28
65	Above average	45	44	38	34	31	27
60		44	43	37	32	30	26
55		42	41	36	31	28	25
50	Average	40	40	34	30	27	24
45		39	37	33	29	26	23
40		38	36	32	28	25	22
35	Below average	37	35	30	27	24	21
30		35	34	29	26	23	20
25		33	32	28	25	22	19
20	Poor	32	30	26	23	20	18
15		20	28	25	22	19	17
10		27	25	24	20	18	16
5	Very poor	24	22	20	18	15	14
0		15	14	12	11	10	10

because this is the recommended HR range (110–150 bpm) for the YMCA cycle ergometer protocol.

The final source of error results from the possibility of a break in linearity of HR and $\dot{V}O_2$ as the values approach maximum. Some individuals may have larger increases in $\dot{V}O_2$ compared to the increase in HR as they approach maximum.

Any and all of these factors may be involved in any submaximal exercise test. The reported SEE for these types of tests has been reported to be as low as ±5% (19) to as high as ±27% (20). Other studies reporting SEE within this range found values of 7% (14), 10%–15% (3), 15% (7), and 15%–16% (9). If a primary goal of the test is obtaining a $\dot{V}O_{2max}$ value to determine a CRF classification, then applying the concepts learned earlier related to the SEE demonstrates a major limitation with this test. Take for example a 30-yr-old woman who completes a submaximal test and has a predicted $\dot{V}O_{2max}$ = 35 mL $\cdot$ kg^{-1} $\cdot$ min^{-1}. This value would suggest that she has "fair" (50th percentile) CRF (see *Table 7.3*). However, when applying the SEE (*e.g.*, use an SEE of ±15% or ±5.25 mL $\cdot$ kg^{-1} $\cdot$ min^{-1}), the resultant predicted $\dot{V}O_{2max}$ range (±2 SEE; 95% confidence interval) would be 24.5–45.5 ml $\cdot$ kg^{-1} $\cdot$ min^{-1}, which would equate to a range from the 3rd percentile to the 92nd percentile ("very poor" to "superior").

Alternatively, if the primary goal of the test is to determine the change in fitness, it is generally accepted that these serial test results may be useful to document change. Certainly, these changes can be observed from the changes in basic test measurements (test time, HR, workload) between the tests. If, for example, the HRs at the same stage of a submaximal exercise test were lower, or if the person were able to perform at a higher workload prior to reaching the test termination criteria (*i.e.*, 70% age-predicted HR$_{max}$), this would indicate improved CRF.

SUMMARY

CRF is an important component of health-related physical fitness and one that is commonly desired by clients. Because the measurement of $\dot{V}O_{2max}$ is limited by factors such as time required, cost, and availability of trained personnel, field tests and submaximal exercise tests are frequently performed. As with other fitness measures obtained via prediction equations, appropriate care is needed in interpreting results when CRF is obtained by an estimation method.

LABORATORY ACTIVITIES

FIELD TEST ASSESSMENTS OF CARDIORESPIRATORY FITNESS

Data Collection
Form groups of three. Each person is required to do the Queens College step test and one of the following field tests to estimate CRF: 1.5-mi run, 12-min run/walk, or 1-mi walk. Follow the instructions for each test provided in this chapter.

Laboratory Report
1. Provide the data collected for each test in a summary table along with calculations to estimate CRF from the two field tests.
2. Provide an interpretation (classification according to *Table 7.3*) of your estimated $\dot{V}O_{2max}$
3. Discuss possible reasons for the differences in CRF estimates between tests.

SUBMAXIMAL EXERCISE TEST ASSESSMENTS OF CARDIORESPIRATORY FITNESS

Data Collection

Form groups of three. One person in the group will do the YMCA cycle test, one person will do the Åstrand-Ryhming cycle, and one person will do the Bruce test. Follow the instructions for each test provided in this chapter.

Laboratory Report

1. Provide the data collected for each test in a summary table along with calculations to estimate CRF from the three tests. Note: You need to perform both the graphing method and the calculation methods to estimate $\dot{V}O_{2max}$.
2. Provide an interpretation (classification according to *Table 7.3*) of your estimated $\dot{V}O_{2max}$.
3. Discuss possible reasons for the differences in CRF estimates between this test and the field tests you performed in the previous lab.
4. Which of the preceding tests do you feel best estimates your fitness level and why?

CASE STUDY

Jen is a 28-yr-old businesswoman who has decided after years of being irregularly active to "get back in shape." Jen ran and played volleyball in high school and remembers doing the 1.5-mi run test in college. She decides to head to the track at the local high school one evening after work to perform the 1.5-mi run test. She arrives at the track, changes into some exercise clothes, and walks a lap to warm up. The temperature is unseasonably warm (86° F with 75% humidity). Jen begins running and feels pretty good for 200 m; however, she begins to have some difficulty breathing because the pace is too fast for her to maintain. After 600 m, Jen starts walking and ends up alternating between running and walking for the rest of the test. Her total test time was 16 min. What would be her predicted $\dot{V}O_{2max}$? Do you think this is an accurate estimate of her $\dot{V}O_{2max}$? What factors, if any, do you think could have contributed to error in the estimation of $\dot{V}O_{2max}$? Do you think this was the best choice of a test for Jen? Explain your answer.

REFERENCES

1. Ainsworth BE, Haskell WL, Whitt MC, et al. Compendium of physical activities: an update of activity codes and MET intensities. *Med Sci Sports Exerc*. 2000;32:S498–516.
2. American College of Sports Medicine position stand. Exercise and hypertension. *MedSci Sports Exerc*. 2004; 36:533–53.
3. Astrand I. Aerobic work capacity in men and women with special reference to age. *Acta Physiol Scand*. 1960;49(suppl 169):1–92.
4. Astrand PO, Rodahl K. *Textbook of Work Physiology*. 3rd ed. New York (NY): McGraw-Hill; 1986. 756 p.
5. Borg G. *Borg's Perceived Exertion and Pain Scales*. Champaign (IL): Human Kinetics; 1998. 104 p.
6. Conley DS, Cureton KJ, Dengel DR, Weyand PG. Validation of the 12-min swim as a field test of peak aerobic power in young men. *Med Sci Sports Exerc*. 1991;23:766–73.
7. Davies CT. Limitations to the prediction of maximum oxygen intake from cardiac frequency measurements. *J Appl Physiol*. 1968;24:700–06.
8. Golding LA, editor. *YMCA Fitness Testing and Assessment Manual*. Champaign (IL): Human Kinetics; 2000. 247 p.
9. Greiwe JS, Kaminsky LA, Whaley MH, Dwyer GD. Evaluation of the ACSM submaximal cycle test for estimating VO_{2max}. *Med Sci Sports Exerc*. 1995;27:1315–20.

10. Kaminsky LA, Wehrli KW, Mahon AD, Robbins GC, Powers DL, Whaley MH. Evaluation of a shallow water running test for the estimation of peak aerobic power. *Med Sci Sports Exerc*. 1993;25:1287–92.

11. Kline G, Porcari JP, Hintermeister R, et al. Estimation of VO_{2max} from a one mile track walk, gender, age and body weight. *Med Sci Sports Exerc*. 1987;19:253.

12. Kodama S, Saito K, Tanaka S, et al. Cardiorespiratory fitness as a quantitative predictor of all-cause mortality and cardiovascular events in healthy men and women; a meta-analysis. *JAMA*. 2009;301(19): 2024–35.

13. Maldonado-Martín S, Brubaker PH, Kaminsky LA, Moore JB, Stewart KP, Kitzman DW. The relationship of six-minute walk to VO_{2peak} and VT in older heart failure patients. *Med Sci Sports Exerc*. 2006;38: 1047–53.

14. Margaria R, Aghemo P, Rovelli E. Indirect determination of maximal O_2 consumption in man. *J Appl Physiol*. 1965;20:1070–73.

15. McArdle WD, Katch FI, Katch VL. *Essentials of Exercise Physiology*. 4th ed. Philadelphia (PA): Lippincott Williams & Wilkins; 2011. 699 p.

16. McArdle WD, Katch FI, Pechar GS, Jacobson L, Ruck S. Reliability and interrelationships between maximal oxygen uptake, physical work capacity and step test scores in college women. *Med Sci Sports*. 1972;4: 182–86.

17. Montoye HJ. The Harvard step test and work capacity. *Rev Can Biol*. 1953;11:491–9.

18. Myers J, Prakash M, Froelicher V, Do D, Partington S, Atwood JE. Exercise capacity and mortality among men referred for exercise testing. *N Engl J Med*. 2002;346(11):793–801.

19. Rowell LB, Taylor HL, Wang Y. Limitations to prediction of maximal oxygen uptake. *J Appl Physiol*. 1964;19:919–27.

20. Storer TW, Davis JA, Caiozzo VJ. Accurate prediction of VO_{2peak} and VT in cycle ergometry. *Med Sci Sports Exerc*. 1990;22:704–12.

21. Tanaka H, Monahan KD, Seals DR. Age-predicted maximal heart rate revisited. *J Am Coll Cardiol*. 20001;37:153–6.

22. Whaley MH, Brubaker PH, Otto RM, American College of Sports Medicine. *ACSM's Guidelines for Exercise Testing and Prescription*. 7th ed. Baltimore (MD): Lippincott Williams & Wilkins; 2005. 366 p.

23. Whaley MH, Kaminsky LA, Dwyer GB, Getchell LH, Norton JA. Predictors of over- and underachievement of age-predicted maximal heart rate. *Med Sci Sports Exerc*. 1992;24:1173–79.

8

Cardiorespiratory Fitness: Maximal Exercise Testing

Why Use Maximal Exercise Tests to Measure Cardiorespiratory Fitness?
Risks
- Contraindications

Monitoring
Personnel
Selecting the Mode for Testing
Protocols
- Bruce Protocol
- Balke-Ware Protocol
- Ball State University/Bruce Ramp Protocol
- Running Protocol
- Cycle Protocols

Test Procedures
- Supervisor
- Test Monitoring Roles

Measured and Estimated $\dot{V}O_{2max}$
- Estimating $\dot{V}O_{2max}$ from Exercise Test Time
- Estimating $\dot{V}O_{2max}$ from Peak Workload

Interpretation
Summary
Laboratory Activities
- Maximal Exercise Tests
  - Data Collection
  - Laboratory Report

Case Study
References

WHY USE MAXIMAL EXERCISE TESTS TO MEASURE CARDIORESPIRATORY FITNESS?

As reviewed in *Chapter 7*, estimates of cardiorespiratory fitness (CRF) can be obtained from submaximal exercise tests. However, maximal exercise tests to determine CRF are preferred when greater accuracy is needed, as is often the case with elite athletes and also in clinical settings where treatment decisions will be influenced by the CRF results. Remember that CRF in combination with other exercise test measurements can provide valuable clinical information, both prognostic and diagnostic, for individuals with and without chronic diseases. This chapter focuses on the procedures used in performing maximal exercise tests in a physical fitness setting primarily for low- and moderate-risk clients. The reader should refer to *Chapter 5* of *ACSM's Guidelines for Exercise Testing and Prescription, Ninth Edition (GETP9)* for more detailed information on performing maximal exercise tests in a clinical setting. An overview of the personnel training requirements for those performing maximal exercise tests is provided in this chapter. Certainly, several factors are involved in determining when it is appropriate to perform a maximal exercise test in a physical fitness versus a clinical setting.

RISKS

Physical activity and exercise are usually associated with positive health outcomes; however, as was discussed in Chapter 2, there are potential risks associated with exercise. In general, the risks associated with exercise increase both with the intensity of exercise and with an increase in client risk classification levels. Thus, maximal exercise testing involves a higher degree of risk than the other health-related physical fitness (HRPF) assessments covered previously in this manual.

ACSM's GETP9 provides a review of the risks associated with exercise and exercise testing. Table 8.1 shows a summary of surveys that have been performed to evaluate the cardiovascular risks and complications that have been documented as occurring with maximal exercise testing. The ACSM's GETP9 also provides a thorough overview of procedures for maximal exercise tests used in clinical settings.

CONTRAINDICATIONS

The risk classification procedures covered in Chapter 2 should be reviewed. Particular attention should be given to Box 2.2, which provides the contraindications for exercise

TABLE 8.1. Cardiac Complications During Exercise Testing[a]

Reference	Year	Site	No. Tests	MI	VF	Death	Hospitalization	Comment
Rochmis (16)	1971	73 U.S. centers	170,000	NA	NA	1	3	34% of tests were symptom limited; 50% of deaths in 8 h; 50% over the next 4 d
Irving (6)	1977	15 Seattle facilities	10,700	NA	4.67	0	NR	
McHenry (10)	1977	Hospital	12,000	0	0	0	0	
Atterhog (1)	1979	20 Swedish centers	50,000	0.8	0.8	6.4	5.2	
Stuart (18)	1980	1,375 U.S. centers	518,448	3.58	4.78	0.5	NR	VF includes other dysrhythmias requiring treatment
Gibbons (4)	1989	Cooper Clinic	71,914	0.56	0.29	0	NR	Only 4% of men and 2% of women had CVD
Knight (9)	1995	Geisinger cardiology service	28,133	1.42	1.77	0	NR	25% were inpatient tests supervised by non-MDs

[a]Events are per 10,000 tests.

MI, myocardial infarction; VF, ventricular fibrillation; NA, not applicable; NR, not reported; CVD, atherosclerotic cardiovascular disease; MD, medical doctor.

From American College of Sports Medicine. ACSM's Guidelines for Exercise Testing and Prescription. 8th ed. Philadelphia (PA): Wolters Kluwer Health Ltd; 2009. 400 p.

testing. It is essential to ensure that the screening process employed rules out the presence of any absolute or relative contraindications prior to allowing the client to perform an exercise test. In a health and fitness setting, any sign or symptom suggestive of underlying disease should be considered a relative contraindication by the health and fitness professional.

MONITORING

The primary outcome measure of a health-related CRF assessment is the measurement of maximal volume of oxygen consumed per unit time ($\dot{V}O_{2max}$). This requires measuring the client's ventilation and the concentrations of O_2 and CO_2 in the inspired and expired air during the maximal exercise test. Although heart rate (HR) is not required to calculate $\dot{V}O_{2max}$, it is typically measured throughout the maximal exercise test. It is also essential to monitor the client for signs and symptoms of exercise intolerance, which would indicate early termination of the test. Indications for terminating the test are provided in *Box 8.1*.

BOX 8.1	Indications for Terminating Exercise Testing

ABSOLUTE INDICATIONS
- Drop in systolic BP of ≥10 mm Hg with an increase in work rate, or if systolic BP decreases below the value obtained in the same position prior to testing when accompanied by other evidence of ischemia
- Moderately severe angina (defined as 3 on standard scale)
- Increasing nervous system symptoms (*e.g.*, ataxia, dizziness, or near syncope)
- Signs of poor perfusion (cyanosis or pallor)
- Technical difficulties monitoring the ECG or SBP
- Subject's desire to stop
- Sustained ventricular tachycardia
- ST elevation (+1.0 mm) in leads without diagnostic Q waves (other than V_1 or aVR)

RELATIVE INDICATIONS
- Drop in systolic BP of ≥10 mm Hg with an increase in work rate, or if systolic BP below the value obtained in the same position prior to testing
- ST or QRS changes such as excessive ST depression (>2 mm horizontal or downsloping ST-segment depression) or marked axis shift
- Arrhythmias other than sustained ventricular tachycardia, including multifocal PVCs, triplets of PVCs, supraventricular tachycardia, heart block, or bradyarrhythmias
- Fatigue, shortness of breath, wheezing, leg cramps, or claudication
- Development of bundle-branch block or intraventricular conduction delay that cannot be distinguished from ventricular tachycardia
- Increasing chest pain
- Hypertensive response (SBP of >250 mm Hg and/or a DBP of >115 mm Hg).

aVR, augmented voltage right; BP, blood pressure; DBP, diastolic blood pressure; ECG, electrocardiogram; PVC, premature ventricular contraction; SBP, systolic blood pressure; V_1, chest lead I.
Reprinted with permission from (5).

TABLE 8.2. Recommendations for the Timing of Monitoring Measures			
Variable	Before Exercise Test	During Exercise Test	After Exercise Test
ECG	Monitored continuously; recorded supine position and posture of exercise	Monitored continuously; recorded during the last 15 s of each stage (interval protocol) or the last 15 s of each 2-min period (ramp protocols)	Monitored continuously; recorded immediately postexercise, during the last 15 s of first min of recovery, and then every 2 min thereafter
HR[b]	Monitored continuously; recorded supine position and posture of exercise	Monitored continuously; recorded during the last 5 s of each min	Monitored continuously; recorded during the last 5 s of each min
BP[a,b]	Measured and recorded in supine position and posture of exercise	Measured and recorded during the last 45 s of each stage (interval protocol) or the last 45 s of each 2-min period (ramp protocols)	Measured and recorded immediately postexercise and then every 2 min thereafter
Signs and symptoms	Monitored continuously; recorded as observed	Monitored continuously; recorded as observed	Monitored continuously; recorded as observed
RPE	Explain scale	Recorded during the last 5 s of each min	Obtain peak exercise value then not measured in recovery
Gas exchange	Baseline reading to assure proper operational status	Measured continuously	Generally not needed in recovery

[a]An unchanged or decreasing systolic blood pressure with increasing workloads should be retaken (*i.e.*, verified immediately).
[b]In addition, BP and HR should be assessed and recorded whenever adverse symptoms or abnormal ECG changes occur.
ECG, electrocardiogram; HR, heart rate; BP, blood pressure; RPE, ratings of perceived exertion.
Reprinted from Brubaker PH, Kaminsky LA, Whaley MH. *Coronary Artery Disease*. Champaign (IL): Human Kinetics; 2002. 182 p.

Maximal exercise tests are also performed in preventative and rehabilitative exercise program settings. Because the opportunity exists to observe a variety of different physiological responses to exercise, additional monitoring including exercise electrocardiography, blood pressure (BP), and measurement of O_2 saturation are routinely performed with the assessment of CRF. The *ACSM's GETP9* provides a thorough overview of the procedures used in clinical exercise testing settings. *Table 8.2* provides recommendations for the timing of monitoring measures for maximal exercise testing. These additional monitoring measures require trained staff and some additional equipment, which are common to most clinical exercise facilities.

PERSONNEL

The *ACSM's GETP9* recommends the following:

In all situations where exercise testing is performed, site personnel should at least be certified at a level of basic life support (CPR) and have automated external defibrillator (AED) training. Preferably, one or more staff members should also be certified in first aid and advanced cardiac life support (ACLS) (8).

This recommendation points out some facility and equipment requirements for laboratories, specifically access to an AED (as shown in *Fig. 8.1*) and first aid equipment. The facility also needs to have a written set of emergency procedures with a regular schedule of review/practice sessions in which all personnel must participate as illustrated in *Figure 8.2*.

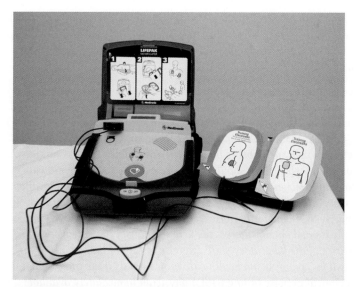

■ **FIGURE 8.1.** An automated external defibrillator is essential in all physical fitness assessment settings. (Photograph by Ball State University.)

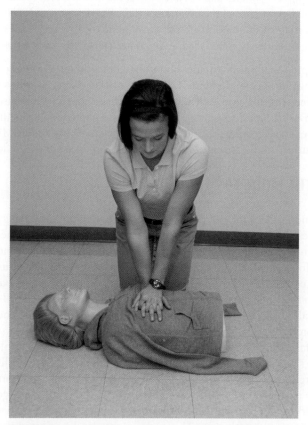

■ **FIGURE 8.2.** Regular emergency procedure drills should include a practice session of cardiopulmonary resuscitation (CPR). (Photograph by Ball State University.)

The guidelines for the recommendations for physician supervision of testing were presented in *Figure 2.4* in *Chapter 2* of this manual. The *ACSM's GETP9* provides the following guidance concerning physician and nonphysician supervision of maximal exercise tests:

> *There is consensus that exercise testing of all patient risk groups can be supervised by nonphysician health care professionals if the professional is specially trained in clinical exercise testing and a physician is immediately available if needed (12). There is also general agreement that such testing in patients at low risk can be supervised by nonphysicians, without a physician being immediately available. There is no consensus as to whether or not nonphysicians should supervise exercise testing in patients at moderate risk without a physician immediately available. Having a physician available for testing of patients at moderate risk is recommended, but whether or not a physician must be immediately available for exercise testing of patients at moderate risk will depend on local policies and circumstances, the health status of the patients, and the training and experience of the laboratory staff. Exercise testing of individuals at high risk can be supervised by nonphysician health care professionals if the professional is specially trained in clinical exercise testing with a physician immediately available if needed. Exercise testing of individuals at moderate risk can be supervised by nonphysician health care professionals if the professional is specially trained in clinical exercise testing, but whether or not a physician must be immediately available for exercise testing is dependent upon local policies and circumstances, the health status of the patients, and the training and experience of the laboratory staff. Physicians responsible for supervising exercise testing should meet or exceed the minimal competencies for supervision and interpretation of results as established by the American Heart Association (17).*

Thus, it is accepted that a trained and experienced health care professional, such as an American College of Sports Medicine (ACSM)-certified exercise professional with the requisite knowledge, skills, and abilities, can administer maximal exercise tests. The job task analysis (JTA) with performance domains and associated job tasks that are required for performing exercise testing are addressed in *Appendix D* of the *ACSM's GETP9*. Also, a list of the cognitive skills required of exercise test supervisors is provided in *Box 8.2*.

SELECTING THE MODE FOR TESTING

The most common modes for exercise testing are the treadmill and the cycle ergometer. These two modes are commonly used because of the ability to easily replicate and control work rates. Arm ergometers, which also have the ability to replicate and control work rates, are used for individuals with disabilities that prevent or limit the use of their legs.

For several reasons, the default, or standard, selection for maximal exercise testing is the treadmill. In the United States, there is more experience with treadmill testing; and for most people, walking is the most common form of daily movement. Generally, treadmill exercise tests produce the higher $\dot{V}O_{2max}$ values than tests on cycle ergometers because the relative unfamiliarity with cycling often results in local fatigue. Unless compelling reasons exist to suggest otherwise, the choice for exercise mode is typically the treadmill.

The cycle ergometer may be the preferred mode in certain situations. If the client were a trained cyclist or desires to exercise primarily on a cycle ergometer, then a cycle test would be appropriate. The principle of specificity, which was discussed in Chapter 5, applies in this situation. The cycle might also be selected if the client has a disability, injury, or health condition that would make walking difficult or that could actually be worsened by walking. Individuals who are obese may be better served by a

---

BOX 8.2   **Cognitive Skills Required to Competently Supervise Exercise Tests**

- Knowledge of appropriate indications for exercise testing
- Knowledge of alternative physiologic cardiovascular tests
- Knowledge of appropriate contraindications, risks, and risk assessment of testing
- Knowledge to promptly recognize and treat complications of exercise testing
- Competence in cardiopulmonary resuscitation and successful completion of an American Heart Association-sponsored course in advance cardiovascular life support and renewal on a regular basis
- Knowledge of various exercise protocols and indications for each
- Knowledge of basic cardiovascular and exercise physiology including hemodynamic response to exercise
- Knowledge of cardiac arrhythmia and the ability to recognize and treat serious arrhythmias (see *Appendix C* within *GETP9*)
- Knowledge of cardiovascular drugs and how they can affect exercise performance, hemodynamics, and the electrocardiogram (see *Appendix A* within *GETP9*)
- Knowledge of the effects of age and disease on hemodynamic and the electrocardiographic response to exercise
- Knowledge of principles and details of exercise testing including proper lead placement and skin preparation
- Knowledge of endpoints of exercise testing and indications to terminate exercise testing

Adapted from (17).

---

cycle that supports body weight (as opposed to the treadmill in which the individual's body must support all weight). Other reasons for selecting a cycle ergometer may be related to facility constraints, such as space and power supply. The cycle ergometer also costs less, is more portable, and operates more quietly than a treadmill.

PROTOCOLS

Once the decision on mode of exercise is made, the testing supervisor needs to determine which test protocol to employ. It is wise to set one standard, or default, protocol that will be used most typically within a given facility. A standard protocol allows for the monitoring of typical, expected responses during the test as well as for comparisons between tests. There are appropriate reasons for altering the standard protocol and some principles that should guide this process. One determining factor is whether the protocol will result in a maximal effort between 6 and 15 min (ideally between 8 and 12 min). A second consideration, applicable only to treadmill tests, is whether the work rate should be increased only through an increase in grade (*i.e.*, a fixed speed protocol) or by increasing both speed and grade. The last consideration is how to increment the work rates, either in stages or as a slow, continuous increase (ramp style).

There are many standardized protocols from which to choose, as indicated in *Figure 8.3*. Some facilities choose to individualize the protocol to reach a target test time associated with a pretest prediction of the client's $\dot{V}O_{2max}$ based on client characteristics. Typically,

FUNCTIONAL CLASS	CLINICAL STATUS	O₂ COST ml/kg/min	METS	BICYCLE ERGOMETER	BRUCE 3 MIN STAGES MPH / %AGR		RAMP PER 30 SEC MPH / %GR	
NORMAL AND I	HEALTHY, DEPENDENT ON AGE, ACTIVITY							
		73.5	21					
		70	20	FOR 70 KG BODY WEIGHT Kpm/min (WATTS)	5.5	20		
		66.5	19					
		63	18					
		59.5	17		5.0	18		
		56.0	16					
		52.5	15					
		49.0	14	1500 (246)	4.2	16	3.0	25.0
		45.5	13				3.0	24.0
							3.0	23.0
		42.0	12	1350 (221)			3.0	22.0
							3.0	21.0
		38.5	11	1200 (197)			3.0	20.0
							3.0	19.0
		35.0	10	1050 (172)	3.4	14	3.0	18.0
							3.0	17.0
		31.5	9	900 (148)			3.0	16.0
							3.0	15.0
		28.0	8				3.0	14.0
				750 (123)			3.0	13.0
	SEDENTARY HEALTHY	24.5	7		2.5	12	3.0	12.0
				600 (98)			3.0	11.0
		21.0	6				3.0	10.0
II				450 (74)			3.0	9.0
	LIMITED	17.5	5				3.0	8.0
							3.0	7.0
		14.0	4	300 (49)	1.7	10	3.0	6.0
III	SYMPTOMATIC						3.0	5.0
		10.5	3	150 (24)			3.0	4.0
							3.0	3.0
		7.0	2				3.0	2.0
							3.0	1.0
							3.0	0
							2.5	0
IV		3.5	1				2.0	0
							1.5	0
							1.0	0
							0.5	0

■ **FIGURE 8.3.** Common exercise protocols and associated metabolic costs of each stage. (Adapted from American College of Sports Medicine. *ACSM's Guidelines for Exercise Testing and Prescription.* 9th ed. Philadelphia [PA]: Lippincott Williams & Wilkins; 2014. p. 124–25.)

TREADMILL PROTOCOLS

BALKE-WARE column note: %GRADE AT 3.3 MPH 1 MIN STAGES

METS	BRUCE RAMP (PER MIN) MPH	%GR	BALKE-WARE	USAFSAM MPH	%GR	"SLOW" USAFSAM MPH	%GR	MODIFIED BALKE MPH	%GR	ACIP MPH	%GR	MOD. NAUGHTON (CHF) MPH	%GR
21	5.8	20											
20	5.6	19											
19													
18	5.3	18											
17	5.0	18											
16	4.8	17											
15			26, 25	3.3	25					3.4	24.0		
14	4.5	16	24, 23										
13	4.2	16	22, 21					3.0	25	3.1	24.0	3.0	25
12	4.1	15	20, 19	3.3	20			3.0	22.5			3.0	22.5
11	3.8	14	18, 17					3.0	20	3.0	21.0	3.0	20
10	3.4	14	16, 15	3.3	15			3.0	17.5	3.0	17.5	3.0	17.5
9	3.1	13	14, 13			2	25	3.0	15	3.0	14.0	3.0	15
8	2.8	12	12, 11	3.3	10	2	20	3.0	12.5			3.0	12.5
7	2.5	12	10, 9			2	15	3.0	10	3.0	10.5	3.0	10
6	2.3	11	8, 7	3.3	5			3.0	7.5	3.0	7.0	3.0	7.5
5	2.1	10	6, 5			2	10	3.0	5			2.0	10.5
4	1.7	10	4, 3			2	5	3.0	2.5	3.0	3.0	2.0	7.0
3	1.3	5	2, 1	3.3	0			3.0	0	2.5	2.0	2.0	3.5
2				2.0	0	2	0	2.0	0	2.0	0.0	1.5	0
1	1.0	0										1.0	0

these individualized protocols are determined by a computer program found on some commercial exercise testing systems. It is beyond the scope of this manual to provide a thorough explanation of many different protocols including arm ergometer protocols; however, the most commonly used protocols that would be applicable to HRPF assessment are reviewed. These include the most frequently used clinical protocol (Bruce), a fixed-speed walking protocol (Balke), a standardized treadmill ramping protocol (Ball State University [BSU]/Bruce), a treadmill running protocol (Costill/Fox), and a cycle protocol.

BRUCE PROTOCOL

Dr. Robert Bruce, a cardiologist, developed the Bruce protocol, which has been used in clinical exercise testing laboratories for approximately 40 yr (3). Surveys of exercise testing laboratories in the United States have consistently reported the Bruce protocol, or modified versions, to be the one most (82%) commonly used (11). This popularity is in part a result of the substantial amount of data on the typical responses expected with the Bruce protocol, including predictions of $\dot{V}O_{2max}$, based on treadmill time, as will be reviewed later in this chapter.

The Bruce protocol consists of 3-min stages, where the speed and grade both increase with each stage, and the work rate increment is approximately 3 metabolic equivalents (METs) per stage. The initial stage of this protocol is set at a MET level of 4.6, which may be too large of a requirement for deconditioned adults, many elderly individuals, and patients with cardiac and pulmonary disease. A modified version of this protocol includes either one or two preliminary stages (stages 0 and 0.5) as shown in *Table 8.3*.

BALKE-WARE PROTOCOL

Another commonly used treadmill protocol is the Balke-Ware, developed by Dr. Bruno Balke and colleagues (2). The main features of this protocol are that it is of fixed speed, and the rate of increment in work rate is relatively small ($\approx$0.5 METs) at each stage (1 min). There have been several modifications made to this protocol, one of which has been employed routinely over the years at the Cooper Clinic in Dallas, Texas, and that has produced the normative chart for interpreting CRF. The original Balke-Ware protocol and some common modifications are shown in *Table 8.4*.

TABLE 8.3. Bruce Treadmill Protocol (3)			
Stage	**Time (min:s)**	**Speed (mph)**	**Grade (%)**
1	0:00	1.7	10.0
2	3:00	2.5	12.0
3	6:00	3.4	14.0
4	9:00	4.2	18.0
5	12:00	5.0	18.0
6	15:00	5.5	20.0
7	18:00	6.0	22.0
Stage	**Time (min:s)**	**Speed (mph)**	**Grade (%)**
0	0:00	1.7	0.0
0.5	3:00	2.5	5.0

See *Figure 8.3* for estimated metabolic equivalent levels. Note: a modification for less fit clients is to add one or two preliminary stages. From (3).

TABLE 8.4. Original and Modifications of the Balke-Ware Treadmill Protocol (2)

	Original				Modified[a]		
Stage	Time (min:s)	Speed (mph)	Grade (%)	Stage	Time (min:s)	Speed (mph)	Grade (%)
1	0:00	3.3	1.0	1	0:00	3.0	0.0
2	1:00	3.3	2.0	2	2:00	3.0	2.5
3	2:00	3.3	3.0	3	4:00	3.0	5.0
4	3:00	3.3	4.0	4	6:00	3.0	7.5
5	4:00	3.3	5.0	5	8:00	3.0	10.0
6	5:00	3.3	6.0	6	10:00	3.0	12.5
7	6:00	3.3	7.0	7	12:00	3.0	15.0
8	7:00	3.3	8.0	8	14:00	3.0	17.5
9	8:00	3.3	9.0	9	16:00	3.0	20.0
10	9:00	3.3	10.0	10	18:00	3.0	22.5
11	10:00	3.3	11.0	11	20:00	3.0	25.0
13	12:00	3.3	13.0				
14	13:00	3.3	14.0				
15	14:00	3.3	15.0				
16	15:00	3.3	16.0				
17	16:00	3.3	17.0				
18	17:00	3.3	18.0				
19	18:00	3.3	19.0				
20	19:00	3.3	20.0				
21	20:00	3.3	21.0				
22	21:00	3.3	22.0				
23	22:00	3.3	23.0				
24	23:00	3.3	24.0				
25	24:00	3.3	25.0				
26	25:00	3.3	26.0				

[a]The speed for the modified protocol can be selected to meet the comfort level of the patient. Other common variations are 2.0 and 2.5 mph. See *Figure 8.3* for estimated metabolic equivalent levels.
From (2).

BALL STATE UNIVERSITY/BRUCE RAMP PROTOCOL

Ramp protocols increase the workload more gradually, usually by shortening the stage time and decreasing the work rate increments. Although ramp protocols for cycle ergometers have been available for a longer period of time, systems to provide ramping increments for treadmills have only been available since the 1990s. Owing to the well-known features of the Bruce protocol, a standardized ramping variation of this protocol was developed. The BSU/Bruce ramp protocol increases the work rate every 20 s (≈ 1 MET $\cdot$ min^{-1}) and has speed and grade settings identical to the Bruce protocol at every 3-min period during the test (7). This test protocol is displayed within *Table 8.5*. Monitoring intervals are typically the same as for the standard Bruce protocol. One beneficial feature of this protocol is the ability of the client to walk for a longer period of time than during the standard Bruce protocol. Clients typically have to start running as they begin stage 4 of the Bruce protocol (minute 9), compared to minute 11 of the BSU/Bruce ramp protocol.

TABLE 8.5. The Ball State University (BSU)/Bruce Treadmill Ramp Protocol (7)

Stage	Time (min:s)	Speed (mph)	Grade (%)	Stage	Time (min:s)	Speed (mph)	Grade (%)
1	0:00	1.7	0.0	33	10:40	4.0	15.2
2	0:20	1.7	1.3	34	11:00	4.1	15.4
3	0:40	1.7	2.5	35	11:20	4.2	15.6
4	1:00	1.7	3.7	36	11:40	4.2	16.0
5	1:20	1.7	5.0	37	12:00	4.3	16.2
6	1:40	1.7	6.2	38	12:20	4.4	16.4
7	2:00	1.7	7.5	39	12:40	4.5	16.6
8	2:20	1.7	8.7	40	13:00	4.6	16.8
9	2:40	1.7	10.0	41	13:20	4.7	17.0
10	3:00	1.8	10.2	42	13:40	4.8	17.2
11	3:20	1.9	10.2	43	14:00	4.9	17.4
12	3:40	2.0	10.5	44	14:20	5.0	17.6
13	4:00	2.1	10.7	45	14:40	5.0	18.0
14	4:20	2.2	10.9	46	15:00	5.1	18.0
15	4:40	2.3	11.2	47	15:20	5.1	18.5
16	5:00	2.4	11.2	48	15:40	5.2	18.5
17	5:20	2.5	11.6	49	16:00	5.2	19.0
18	5:40	2.5	12.0	50	16:20	5.3	19.0
19	6:00	2.6	12.2	51	16:40	5.3	19.5
20	6:20	2.7	12.4	52	17:00	5.4	19.5
21	6:40	2.8	12.7	53	17:20	5.4	20.0
22	7:00	2.9	12.9	54	17:40	5.5	20.0
23	7:20	3.0	13.1	55	18:00	5.6	20.0
24	7:40	3.1	13.4	56	18:20	5.6	20.5
25	8:00	3.2	13.6	57	18:40	5.7	20.5
26	8:20	3.3	13.8	58	19:00	5.7	21.0
27	8:40	3.4	14.0	59	19:20	5.8	21.0
28	9:00	3.5	14.2	60	19:40	5.8	21.5
29	9:20	3.6	14.4	61	20:00	5.9	21.5
30	9:40	3.7	14.6	62	20:20	5.9	22.0
31	10:00	3.8	14.8	63	20:40	6.0	22.0
32	10:20	3.9	15.0				

From (7).

RUNNING PROTOCOL

As the principle of specificity would suggest, trained endurance runners will perform best on a protocol that allows them to run at faster speeds and lower elevations than the treadmill tests described earlier. Obviously, because of the increased noise and body motion associated with running protocols, the ability to obtain and monitor variables such as BP and heart function, with the use of an electrocardiogram (ECG), will

TABLE 8.6. Modified Costill/Fox Running Protocol (19)

Stage	Time (min)	Speed (km · h⁻¹)	Grade (%)
Warm-up	0–4	5.0	0.0
Speed increasing stages[a]	4 each	9.5	0.0
		12.0	
		13.5	
		16.0	
Grade increasing stages	2 each		2.0
			4.0
			6.0
			8.0

[a]Speed (4 min per stage) continues to increase until the subject reaches a rating of perceived exertion (RPE) of 13. Then speed remains constant, and the grade increases by 2% every 2 min until exhaustion.
Speeds in mph are 3.1 (warm-up), and 5.9, 7.5, 8.4, and 9.9 (each running speed, respectively).
From (19).

be limited. Thus, these types of protocols are only indicated for low-risk individuals who regularly train for endurance by running. The protocols typically feature a beginning phase where the client runs at a moderate pace for a couple of minutes to warm up, followed by a rapid increase to the peak sustained running speed desired by the client. Further increments in work are obtained by making modest increases in grade until the client reaches maximum capacity. A modified Costill/Fox protocol is shown in *Table 8.6* (19).

CYCLE PROTOCOLS

A cycling protocol involves a non–weight-bearing mode of exercise, and thus the workload is set by pedaling against an external resistance. The ability to push this resistance will be determined to a large degree by the amount of muscle mass a person possesses. Although the absolute level of work will be greater for the larger person, CRF is measured in units relative to body weight (*i.e.*, mL · kg⁻¹ · min⁻¹). *Table 8.7* shows one commonly used protocol for cycle testing, which uses 2-min stages with work rate increments of 150 kg · m · min⁻¹. When testing a larger person, the protocol may start with a higher workload or it may use larger increments during the test.

TABLE 8.7. An Example of a Cycle Test Protocol

Stage	Time (min:s)	Work Rate (kg · m · min⁻¹)
1	0:00	150
2	2:00	300
3	4:00	450
4	6:00	600
5	8:00	750
6	10:00	900
7	12:00	1,050
8	14:00	1,200

Note: For larger individuals, the work rates may need to be doubled.

Ramp protocols are quite popular for cycle ergometry testing. As noted earlier, commercial exercise testing systems will commonly provide a program to develop the ramping protocols.

TEST PROCEDURES

Multiple personnel are needed to administer maximal exercise testing, with the exact number being determined by the amount of monitoring used. A list of the primary job responsibilities is provided in the following text, with modifications made to reduce the number of staff if less monitoring is performed or if the staff are very experienced and can perform multiple responsibilities during a test.

SUPERVISOR

The person acting as test supervisor will have performed a pretest review of the client's risk classification screening information, making sure there are no contraindications for testing. The informed consent document is reviewed again (Note: This would have already been completed at the risk classification screening), and the exercise test procedures are outlined. The supervisor should ensure the client understands that although the objective is to work to a maximal effort level, the test can be stopped at any time, and the staff should be promptly informed if anything unusual is experienced during the test (particularly symptoms of ischemia such as chest discomfort). An explanation of the rating of perceived exertion (RPE) scale should be provided at this time. The supervisor may also perform one of the test technician roles during the test.

TEST MONITORING ROLES

The most commonly monitored variables during a maximal exercise test are the ECG or other measure of HR, metabolic measurements, BP, RPE, and possibly O_2 saturation. Additionally, the treadmill or cycle ergometer work rates need to be controlled by the staff or monitored by the staff if controlled by a computer program.

The protocol should start with a brief 1- to 2-min warm-up (treadmill — slow speed of walking; cycle — unloaded pedaling). During this time, the staff should be making sure all equipment is functioning properly and the client is relatively comfortable on the exercise ergometer. When the staff and the client are ready, the protocol begins and the sequence of measures as described in *Table 8.2* is performed. To ensure client safety, it is important that all staff observes the client during the test and that one specific staff member is assigned this responsibility as a primary role. In many laboratories, the technician performing the BP measurements will also obtain measures of RPE and become the primary observer and communicator with the client. One staff member is typically in charge of recording data (HR, BP, RPE, symptoms) during the test. The technician monitoring the ECG, or other monitor of HR, commonly performs this duty. Also, one technician monitors the readings from the metabolic measurements and can control the workload changes during the test. This technician would also be responsible for the pretest calibration of the metabolic cart and the posttest cleaning and sterilization of the mouthpiece and breathing valve used by the client. The staff should provide feedback to the client throughout the test and encourage a maximal effort. Common objective indicators of maximal effort are a respiratory exchange ratio of ≥ 1.1, a plateau in volume of oxygen consumed per unit time ($\dot{V}O_2$) (no further increase in $\dot{V}O_2$ with an increase in work rate), and achievement of age-predicted maximal HR (HR_{max}). Subjective indicators include an RPE between 17 and 19 and the client's appearance of exhaustion (15).

MEASURED AND ESTIMATED $\dot{V}O_{2max}$

To provide the gold standard measure of CRF, the maximal exercise test must include the assessment of $\dot{V}O_2$ with a metabolic measurement system. These systems will provide measures of exercise ventilation and expired concentrations of O_2 and CO_2 to derive the measurement of $\dot{V}O_2$. These metabolic measurement systems can also provide a detailed recording of the responses throughout the test and can be used to provide other data of interest to the client (*e.g.*, ventilatory threshold).

The measurement of $\dot{V}O_2$ is not always feasible because metabolic measurement systems are relatively expensive to purchase and to maintain. These systems also require additional expertise of the personnel operating them and interpreting results. When direct measurement is not available, it is possible to predict $\dot{V}O_{2max}$ from either the total time or the peak workload obtained during a maximal exercise test. As with all predicted results, interpretation must include an expression of the error range.

ESTIMATING $\dot{V}O_{2max}$ FROM EXERCISE TEST TIME

Several research reports have provided regression equations to obtain an estimate of $\dot{V}O_{2max}$ from exercise test duration. When using prediction models, it is essential that the identical protocol is followed for the test, and that the subjects are not allowed to use handrail support during the treadmill test. It is also desirable to match the characteristics of the subject to the general characteristics of the population that was assessed in the original study. *Table 8.8* provides prediction equations for the Bruce, BSU/Bruce ramp, and Balke-Ware protocols. Note that the standard error of estimates (SEEs) range from ±2.7 to ±4.7 mL $\cdot$ kg^{-1} $\cdot$ min^{-1}. The reference tables for CRF interpretation (*Table 8.9*) also provide an estimate for the modified Balke-Ware protocol used at the Cooper Clinic.

ESTIMATING $\dot{V}O_{2max}$ FROM PEAK WORKLOAD

Another approach to obtaining an estimate of $\dot{V}O_{2max}$ is to use the ACSM metabolic calculations, which can be found in Chapter 7. This method is not desirable because the metabolic calculation equations were developed for steady-state submaximal

TABLE 8.8. Prediction of $\dot{V}O_{2max}$ from Treadmill Test Time			
Source	**Protocol**	**Subject Sample**	**Equation**
Bruce (3)	Bruce	Healthy persons	$\dot{V}O_{2max}$ (mL $\cdot$ kg^{-1} $\cdot$ min^{-1}) = 6.7 − 2.82 (men = 1, women = 2) + 0.056 (time in seconds)
Unpublished Data — Ball State University (BSU) Adult Physical Fitness Program	Bruce	Men and women (N = 296)	$\dot{V}O_{2max}$ (mL $\cdot$ kg^{-1} $\cdot$ min^{-1}) = 3.814 (time in minutes) − 3.938 ± 4.68 (r = 0.87)
Kaminsky (7)	BSU/Bruce ramp protocol	Men and women (N = 392)	$\dot{V}O_{2max}$ (mL $\cdot$ kg^{-1} $\cdot$ min^{-1}) = 3.9 (time in minutes) − 7.0 ± 3.4 (r = 0.93)
Pollock (14)	Balke 3.0 mph	Women (N = 49)	$\dot{V}O_{2max}$ (mL $\cdot$ kg^{-1} $\cdot$ min^{-1}) = 0.023 (time in seconds) + 5.2 ± 2.7 (r = 0.94)
Pollock (13)	Balke 3.3 mph	Men (N = 51)	$\dot{V}O_{2max}$ (mL $\cdot$ kg^{-1} $\cdot$ min^{-1}) = 1.444 (time in minutes) + 14.99 ± 0.025 (r = 0.92)

$\dot{V}O_{2max}$, maximal volume of oxygen consumed per unit time.

work rates. However, for cycle testing or other treadmill protocols without prediction equations based on test time, they are sometimes used.

INTERPRETATION

As with other measures of HRPF, no national standard has been developed and accepted for interpreting CRF. However, the ACSM has long used the data developed by the Cooper Clinic in Dallas, Texas as a source for providing interpretations of CRF assessments. These CRF gender-specific charts are provided in *Table 8.9*. Similar to the body composition norms, it is important to recognize that these values are based on the population that has received these measures and are expressed as percentiles, which may limit their usefulness for interpreting test results from populations with different characteristics.

SUMMARY

The gold standard measure of CRF is the maximal exercise test with measurement of ventilation and the concentrations of O_2 and CO_2 in the inspired and expired air. Because of the increased risks for the client to perform this test, the relatively expensive equipment required to obtain the necessary measurements, and the high level of training required of the testing personnel, this procedure is not routinely performed in all HRPF assessment settings. However, fitness professionals working in preventative and rehabilitative exercise programs will often be involved in performing this form of assessment of CRF.

LABORATORY ACTIVITIES

MAXIMAL EXERCISE TESTS

Data Collection
The class will perform three maximal exercise tests, one each on three different subjects. One student will perform a BSU/Bruce treadmill protocol, one student will perform a modified Costill/Fox running protocol, and one student will perform a maximal test on a cycle ergometer. Follow the instructions for monitoring and test administration presented in this chapter. For each test, a different group of students will perform the roles of the different technicians.

Laboratory Report
1. Using the exercise test data recording sheet (p. 167), make a graph for each test of the HR (x-axis) and $\dot{V}O_2$ (y-axis) relationship.
2. Did all subjects reach a true $\dot{V}O_{2max}$? What objective criteria indicate they did or did not give a maximal effort? Interpret the test results for each subject.
3. For the cycle test, pretend the test was stopped after the subject completed two stages with HR values between 110 and 150 beats per minute (bpm). Use those submaximal data to predict $\dot{V}O_{2max}$ using the methods discussed in *Chapter 7*. How does this predicted value compare to the measured value from the maximal exercise test?
4. Use the prediction formula based on treadmill test time for the BSU/Bruce ramp test to predict $\dot{V}O_{2max}$. How does this predicted value compare to the measured value from the maximal exercise test?
5. Which submaximal assessment (performed by these subjects in the labs from *Chapter 7*) predicted actual $\dot{V}O_{2max}$ the best for each subject? Discuss why this particular submaximal test may have been a better predictor than the other tests for that subject.

TABLE 8.9. Fitness Categories for Maximal Aerobic Power for Men and Women by Age

		MEN							
		Age 20–29				Age 30–39			
%		Balke Treadmill (time)	Max $\dot{V}O_2$ (mL/kg/min)	12-Min Run (miles)	1.5-Mi Run (time)	Balke Treadmill (time)	Max $\dot{V}O_2$ (mL/kg/min)	12-Min Run (miles)	1.5-Mi Run (time)
99	Superior	31:30	60.5	2.00	8:29	30:00	58.3	1.94	8:49
95		28:05	55.5	1.86	9:17	27:03	54.1	1.82	9:33
90		27:00	54.0	1.81	9:34	25:25	51.7	1.75	10:01
85	Excellent	25:30	51.8	1.75	10:00	24:13	50.0	1.70	10:24
80		25:00	51.1	1.73	10:09	23:06	48.3	1.66	10:46
75		23:13	48.5	1.66	10:43	22:10	47.0	1.62	11:06
70	Good	22:30	47.5	1.63	10:59	21:30	46.0	1.59	11:22
65		22:00	46.8	1.61	11:10	21:00	45.3	1.57	11:33
60		21:10	45.6	1.58	11:29	20:09	44.1	1.54	11:54
55		21:40	44.8	1.56	11:41	20:00	43.9	1.53	11:58
50	Fair	20:00	43.9	1.53	11:58	19:00	42.4	1.49	12:24
45		19:08	42.6	1.50	12:20	18:07	41.2	1.46	12:50
40		18:30	41.7	1.47	12:38	17:49	40.7	1.44	12:58
35		18:00	41.0	1.45	12:53	17:00	39.5	1.41	13:24
30	Poor	17:17	39.9	1.42	13:15	16:24	38.7	1.39	13:44
25		16:38	39.0	1.40	13:36	15:46	37.8	1.36	14:05
20		15:56	38.0	1.37	14:00	15:00	36.7	1.33	14:34
15		15:00	36.7	1.33	14:34	14:02	35.2	1.29	15:13
10	Very poor	13:37	34.7	1.28	15:30	13:00	33.8	1.25	15:57
5		11:38	31.8	1.20	17:04	11:15	31.2	1.18	17:25
1		8:00	26.5	1.05	20:58	8:00	26.5	1.05	20:58
		$n = 2,328$				$n = 12,730$			

Total $n = 15,058$

(continued)

TABLE 8.9. Fitness Categories for Maximal Aerobic Power for Men and Women by Age (Continued)

MEN

%		Age 40–49				Age 50–59			
		Balke Treadmill (time)	Max VO$_2$ (mL/kg/min)	12-Min Run (miles)	1.5-Mi Run (time)	Balke Treadmill (time)	Max VO$_2$ (mL/kg/min)	12-Min Run (miles)	1.5-Mi Run (time)
99	Superior	28:30	56.1	1.87	9:10	27:00	54.0	1.81	9:34
95		26:00	52.5	1.77	9:51	23:32	49.0	1.68	10:37
90		24:00	49.6	1.69	10:28	22:00	46.8	1.61	11:10
85	Excellent	23:00	48.2	1.65	10:48	20:30	44.6	1.55	11:45
80		21:45	46.4	1.60	11:15	19:37	43.3	1.52	12:08
75		20:42	44.9	1.56	11:40	18:35	41.8	1.48	12:36
70	Good	20:01	43.9	1.53	11:58	18:00	41.0	1.45	12:53
65		19:30	43.1	1.51	12:11	17:08	39.7	1.42	13:20
60		19:00	42.4	1.49	12:24	16:39	39.0	1.40	13:35
55		18:00	41.0	1.45	12:53	16:00	38.1	1.37	13:58
50	Fair	17:22	40.1	1.43	13:12	15:18	37.1	1.34	14:23
45		17:00	39.5	1.41	13:24	15:00	36.7	1.33	14:34
40		16:14	38.4	1.38	13:50	14:12	35.5	1.30	15:06
35		15:38	37.6	1.36	14:11	13:43	34.8	1.28	15:26
30	Poor	15:00	36.7	1.33	14:34	13:00	33.8	1.25	15:58
25		14:30	35.9	1.31	14:53	12:21	32.8	1.23	16:28
20		13:45	34.8	1.28	15:24	11:45	32.0	1.20	16:58
15		13:00	33.8	1.25	15:58	11:00	30.9	1.17	17:38
10	Very poor	12:00	32.3	1.21	16:46	10:00	29.4	1.13	18:37
5		10:01	29.4	1.13	18:48	8:15	26.9	1.06	20:38
1		7:00	25.1	1.01	22:22	5:25	22.8	0.95	25:00
		$n = 18,104$				$n = 10,627$			

Total $n = 28,731$

		MEN							
		Age 60-69				Age 70-79			
%		Balke Treadmill (time)	Max $\dot{V}O_2$ (mL/kg/min)	12-Min Run (miles)	1.5-Mi Run (time)	Balke Treadmill (time)	Max $\dot{V}O_2$ (mL/kg/min)	12-Min Run (miles)	1.5-Mi Run (time)
99	Superior	25:00	51.1	1.73	10:09	24:00	49.6	1.69	10:28
95	Superior	21:18	45.7	1.59	11:26	20:00	43.9	1.53	11:58
90		19:10	42.7	1.50	12:20	17:00	39.5	1.41	13:24
85	Excellent	18:01	41.0	1.45	12:53	16:00	38.1	1.37	13:58
80		17:01	39.6	1.41	13:23	15:00	36.7	1.33	14:34
75		16:09	38.3	1.38	13:52	14:01	35.2	1.29	15:14
70	Good	15:30	37.4	1.35	14:16	13:05	33.9	1.26	15:54
65		15:00	36.7	1.33	14:34	12:32	33.1	1.23	16:19
60		14:15	35.6	1.30	15:04	12:03	32.4	1.21	16:43
55		13:47	34.9	1.28	15:23	11:29	31.6	1.19	17:12
50	Fair	13:02	33.8	1.25	15:56	11:00	30.9	1.17	17:38
45		12:30	33.0	1.23	16:21	10:26	30.1	1.15	18:11
40		12:00	32.3	1.21	16:46	10:00	29.4	1.13	18:38
35		11:30	31.6	1.19	17:11	9:17	28.4	1.10	19:24
30	Poor	10:57	30.8	1.17	17:41	9:00	28.0	1.09	19:43
25		10:04	29.5	1.13	18:33	8:17	26.9	1.06	20:36
20		9:30	28.7	1.11	19:10	7:24	25.7	1.03	21:47
15		8:30	27.3	1.07	20:19	6:40	24.6	1.00	22:52
10	Very poor	7:21	25.6	1.03	21:51	5:31	23.0	0.95	24:49
5		5:57	23.6	0.97	24:03	4:00	20.8	0.89	27:58
1		3:16	19.7	0.86	29:47	2:15	18.2	0.82	32:46
		$n = 2,971$				$n = 417$			

Total $n = 3,388$

(continued)

TABLE 8.9. Fitness Categories for Maximal Aerobic Power for Men and Women by Age *(Continued)*

WOMEN

%		Age 20–29				Age 30–39		
		Balke Treadmill (time)	Max V̇O₂ (mL/kg/min)	12-Min Run (miles)	1.5-Mi Run (time)	Balke Treadmill (time)	Max V̇O₂ (mL/kg/min)	12-Min Run (miles)	1.5-Mi Run (time)

%		Balke Treadmill (time)	Max V̇O₂ (mL/kg/min)	12-Min Run (miles)	1.5-Mi Run (time)	Balke Treadmill (time)	Max V̇O₂ (mL/kg/min)	12-Min Run (miles)	1.5-Mi Run (time)
99	Superior	27:23	54.5	1.83	9:30	25:37	52.0	1.76	9:58
95		24:00	49.6	1.69	10:28	22:26	47.4	1.63	11:00
90		22:00	46.8	1.61	11:10	21:00	45.3	1.57	11:33
85	Excellent	21:00	45.3	1.57	11:33	20:00	43.9	1.53	11:58
80		20:01	43.9	1.53	11:58	19:00	42.4	1.49	12:24
75		19:00	42.4	1.49	12:24	18:02	41.0	1.45	12:53
70	Good	18:04	41.1	1.46	12:51	17:01	39.6	1.41	13:24
65		18:00	41.0	1.45	12:53	16:18	38.5	1.38	13:47
60		17:00	39.5	1.41	13:24	15:43	37.7	1.36	14:08
55		16:17	38.5	1.38	13:48	15:10	36.9	1.34	14:28
50	Fair	15:50	37.8	1.37	14:04	15:00	36.7	1.33	14:34
45		15:00	36.7	1.33	14:34	14:00	35.2	1.29	15:14
40		14:36	36.1	1.32	14:50	13:20	34.2	1.27	15:43
35		14:00	35.2	1.29	15:14	13:00	33.8	1.25	15:58
30	Poor	13:15	34.1	1.26	15:46	12:03	32.4	1.21	16:42
25		12:30	33.0	1.23	16:21	11:47	32.0	1.20	16:56
20		12:00	32.3	1.21	16:46	11:00	30.9	1.17	17:38
15		11:01	30.9	1.17	17:38	10:00	29.4	1.13	18:37
10	Very poor	10:04	29.5	1.13	18:33	9:00	28.0	1.09	19:43
5		8:43	27.6	1.08	20:03	7:33	25.9	1.03	21:34
1		6:00	23.7	0.97	23:58	5:27	22.9	0.95	24:56
		n = 1,280				*n* = 4,257			

Total *n* = 5,537

WOMEN

%	Category	Age 40-49				Age 50-59			
		Balke Treadmill (time)	Max $\dot{V}O_2$ (mL/kg/min)	12-Min Run (miles)	1.5-Mi Run (time)	Balke Treadmill (time)	Max $\dot{V}O_2$ (mL/kg/min)	12-Min Run (miles)	1.5-Mi Run (time)
99	Superior	25:00	51.1	1.73	10:09	21:31	46.1	1.59	11:20
95	Superior	21:00	45.3	1.57	11:33	18:01	41.0	1.45	12:53
90	Excellent	19:30	43.1	1.51	12:11	16:30	38.8	1.39	13:40
85	Excellent	18:02	41.0	1.45	12:53	15:16	37.0	1.34	14:24
80	Excellent	17:02	39.6	1.41	13:23	15:00	36.7	1.33	14:34
75	Good	16:22	38.6	1.39	13:45	14:02	35.2	1.29	15:13
70	Good	16:00	38.1	1.37	13:58	13:20	34.2	1.27	15:43
65	Good	15:01	36.7	1.33	14:34	12:40	33.3	1.24	16:13
60	Good	14:30	35.9	1.31	14:53	12:13	32.6	1.22	16:35
55	Fair	14:01	35.2	1.29	15:13	12:00	32.3	1.21	16:46
50	Fair	13:32	34.5	1.27	15:34	11:21	31.4	1.19	17:19
45	Fair	13:00	33.8	1.25	15:58	11:00	30.9	1.17	17:38
40	Fair	12:18	32.8	1.22	16:31	10:19	29.9	1.14	18:18
35	Poor	12:00	32.3	1.21	16:46	10:00	29.4	1.13	18:37
30	Poor	11:10	31.1	1.18	17:29	9:30	28.7	1.11	19:10
25	Poor	10:32	30.2	1.15	18:05	9:00	28.0	1.09	19:43
20	Poor	10:00	29.4	1.13	18:37	8:10	26.8	1.06	20:44
15	Very poor	9:07	28.2	1.10	19:35	7:30	25.8	1.03	21:38
10	Very poor	8:04	26.6	1.05	20:52	6:40	24.6	1.00	22:52
5	Very poor	7:00	25.1	1.01	22:22	5:33	23.0	0.95	24:46
1	Very poor	5:00	22.2	0.93	25:49	3:31	20.1	0.87	29:09

$n = 5,908$

$n = 3,923$

Total $n = 9,831$

(continued)

TABLE 8.9. Fitness Categories for Maximal Aerobic Power for Men and Women by Age (*Continued*)

WOMEN

%		Age 60-69 Balke Treadmill (time)	Max $\dot{V}O_2$ (mL/kg/min)	12-Min Run (miles)	1.5-Mi Run (time)	Age 70-79 Balke Treadmill (time)	Max $\dot{V}O_2$ (mL/kg/min)	12-Min Run (miles)	1.5-Mi Run (time)
99	Superior	19:00	42.4	1.49	12:24	19:00	42.4	1.49	12:24
95		15:46	37.8	1.36	14:05	15:21	37.2	1.35	14:21
90		14:30	35.9	1.31	14:53	12:06	32.5	1.22	16:40
85	Excellent	13:17	34.2	1.26	15:45	12:00	32.3	1.21	16:46
80		12:15	32.7	1.22	16:33	10:47	30.6	1.16	17:51
75		12:00	32.3	1.21	16:46	10:16	29.8	1.14	18:21
70	Good	11:09	31.1	1.18	17:30	10:01	29.4	1.13	18:37
65		11:00	30.9	1.17	17:38	10:00	29.4	1.13	18:37
60		10:10	29.7	1.14	18:27	9:06	28.1	1.10	19:36
55		10:00	29.4	1.13	18:37	9:00	28.0	1.09	19:43
50	Fair	9:35	28.8	1.12	19:04	8:44	27.6	1.08	20:02
45		9:07	28.2	1.10	19:35	8:05	26.7	1.05	20:52
40		8:33	27.3	1.07	20:16	7:35	25.9	1.03	21:31
35		8:04	26.6	1.05	20:52	7:07	25.3	1.02	22:07
30	Poor	7:32	25.9	1.03	21:36	6:44	24.7	1.00	22:46
25		7:01	25.1	1.01	22:21	6:23	24.2	0.99	23:20
20		6:39	24.6	1.00	22:52	5:55	23.5	0.97	24:06
15		6:12	23.9	0.98	23:37	5:00	22.2	0.93	25:49
10	Very poor	5:32	23.0	0.95	24:48	4:30	21.5	0.91	26:51
5		4:45	21.8	0.92	26:19	3:12	19.6	0.86	30:00
1		3:07	19.5	0.86	30:12	1:17	16.8	0.78	36:13

n = 1,131   *n* = 155

Total *n* = 1,286

Adapted with permission from *Physical Fitness Assessments and Norms for Adults and Law Enforcement*. The Cooper Institute, Dallas, Texas. 2009. For more information: www.cooperinstitute.org

CASE STUDY

Marge is a 42-yr-old sedentary woman who came to the ABC Fitness Club to have her CRF measured. She chose to have a maximal exercise test done to measure her $\dot{V}O_{2max}$. The testing supervisor selected the standard Bruce protocol for the test, and Marge completed 6 min and 42 s before she signaled that she needed to stop the exercise test. Her measured HR_{max} was 183 bpm, and she rated her RPE as 19. Unfortunately, there were technical problems with the metabolic cart and no data were available. Can you provide a prediction of Marge's $\dot{V}O_{2max}$ based on the exercise test data? If so, how would you interpret the $\dot{V}O_{2max}$? Do you agree that this was the best protocol for Marge? If so, explain why. If not, which protocol would you have selected, and why would you have selected this alternate protocol?

REFERENCES

1. Atterhog JH, Jonsson B, Samuelsson R. Exercise testing: a prospective study of complication rates. *Am Heart J.* 1979;98:572–79.
2. Balke B, Ware R. An experimental study of physical fitness of Air Force personnel. *U S Armed Forces Med J.* 1959;10:675–88.
3. Bruce RA, Hosmer F, Kusumi F. Maximal oxygen intake and nomographic assessment of functional aerobic impairment in cardiovascular disease. *Am Heart J.* 1973;85:546–62.
4. Gibbons L, Blair SN, Kohl HW, Cooper K. The safety of maximal exercise testing. *Circulation.* 1989;80:846–52.
5. Gibbons RJ, Balady GJ, Bricker JT, et al. Committee to Update the 1997 Exercise Testing Guidelines. ACC/AHA 2002 guideline update for exercise testing: summary article. A report of the American College of Cardiology/American Heart Association Task Force on Practice Guidelines (Committee to Update the 1997 Exercise Testing Guidelines). *J Am Coll Cardiol.* 2002;40(8):1531–40.
6. Irving JB, Bruce RA, DeRouen TA. Variations in and significance of systolic pressure during maximal exercise (treadmill) testing. *Am J Cardiol.* 1977;39:841–48.
7. Kaminsky LA, Whaley MH. Evaluation of a new standardized ramp protocol: the BSU/Bruce Ramp protocol. *J Cardiopulm Rehabil.* 1998;18:438–44.
8. Kern KB, Halperin JR, Field J. New Guidelies for cardiopulmonary resuscitation and emergency cardiac care: changes in the management of cardiac arrest. *JAMA.* 2001;285(10):1267–9.
9. Knight JA, Laubach CA Jr, Butcher RJ, Menapace FJ. Supervision of clinical exercise testing by exercise physiologists. *Am J Cardiol.* 1995;75(5):390–91.
10. McHenry PL. Risks of graded exercise testing. *Am J Cardiol.* 1977;39(6):935–37.
11. Myers J, Arena R, Franklin B, et al. Recommendations for clinical exercise laboratories: a scientific statement from the American Heart Association. *Circulation.* 2009;119(24):3144–61.
12. Myers JN, Voodi L, Froelicher VF. A survey of exercise testing: methods, utilization, interpretation, and safety in the VAHCS. *Med Sci Sports Exerc.* 2000;32:S143.
13. Pollock ML, Bohannon RL, Cooper KH, et al. A comparative analysis of four protocols for maximal treadmill stress testing. *Am Heart J.* 1976;92:39–46.
14. Pollock ML, Foster C, Schmidt D, Hellman C, Linnerud AC, Ward A. Comparative analysis of physiologic responses to three different maximal graded exercise test protocols in healthy women. *Am Heart J.* 1982;103:363–73.
15. Pollock ML, Wilmore JH. *Exercise in Health and Disease: Evaluation and Prescription for Prevention and Rehabilitation.* 2nd ed. Philadelphia (PA): WB Saunders; 1990. 741 p.
16. Rochmis P, Blackburn H. Exercise tests. A survey of procedures, safety, and litigation experience in approximately 170,000 tests. *JAMA.* 1971;217(8):1061–66.
17. Rodgers GP, Ayaian JZ, Balady G, et al. American College of Cardiology/American Heart Association Clinical Competence Statement on Stress Testing. A Report of the College of Cardiology/American Heart Association/American College of Physicians-American Society of Internal Medicine Task Force on Clinical Competence. *Circulation.* 2000;102(14):1726–38.
18. Stuart RJ, Ellestad MH. National survey of exercise stress testing facilities. *Chest.* 1980;77(1):94–7.
19. Trappe SW, Costill DL, Vukovich MD, Jones J, Melham T. Aging among elite distance runners: a 22-yr longitudinal study. *J Appl Physiol.* 1996;80:285–90.

A

Conversions

Length or Height

1 kilometer = 1,000 meters (m)

1 kilometer = 0.62137 miles

1 mile = 1,609.35 meters

1 meter = 100 centimeters (cm) = 1,000 millimeters (mm)

1 foot = 0.3048 meters

1 meter = 3.281 feet = 39.37 inches

1 inch = 2.54 centimeters

0.394 inches = 1 centimeter

Mass or Weight

1 kilogram = 1,000 grams (g) = 10 Newtons (N)

1 kilogram = 2.2 pounds

1 pound = 0.454 kilograms

1 gram = 1,000 milligrams (mg)

1 pound = 453.592 grams

1 ounce = 28.3495 grams

1 gram = 0.035 ounces

Volume

1 liter = 1,000 milliliters (mL)

1 liter = 1.05 quarts

1 quart = 0.9464 liters

1 milliliter = 1 cubic centimeter (cc or cm^3)

1 gallon = 3.785 liters (L)

Work

1 Newton-meter = 1 Joule (J)

1 Newton-meter = 0.7375 foot-pounds

1 foot-pound = 1.36 Newton-meters

1 kiloJoule (1,000 J) = 0.234 kilocalories (kcal)

1 foot-pound = 0.1383 kilograms per meter (kg · m^{-1})

1 kg · m^{-1} = 7.23 foot-pounds

Velocity

1 meter per second (m · s⁻¹) = 2.2372 miles per hour (mph)

1 mile per hour = 26.8 meters per minute
(m · min⁻¹) = 1.6093 kilometers per hour (kph)

Power

1 kilogram-meter per minute (kg · m⁻¹ · min⁻¹) = 0.1635 watts (W)

1 watt = 6.12 kg · m⁻¹ · min⁻¹

1 kg · m⁻¹ · min⁻¹ = 1 kp · m⁻¹ · min⁻¹

1 watt = 1 Joule per second (J · s⁻¹)

1 horsepower (hp) = 745.7 watts

Temperature

1° C = 1° Kelvin (K) = 1.8° F

1° F = 0.56° C

Metric Roots

deci = 1/10

centi = 1/100

milli = 1/1,000

kilo = 1,000

B

Forms[1]

Risk Stratification Assessment
Body Composition Data Form
Muscular Fitness Data Form
Flexibility Data Form
Submaximal Cycle Test Data Form
Exercise Test Data Form

---

[1]All forms used with the permission of the Ball State University Clinical Exercise Physiology Program.

RISK STRATIFICATION ASSESSMENT

NAME: _____   Test Date: _____   AGE: _____   GENDER (circle one)   M   F

Age	Yes	No				
Family History	Yes	No	If yes, who/what _____			
Cigarette Smoker	Yes	No				
Hypertension	Yes	No	Resting BP _____ mmHg	Medication	Yes	No
Hypercholesterolemia	Yes	No	LDL ____ mg · dL^{-1} HDL ____ mg · dL^{-1}	Medication	Yes	No
Impaired Fasting Glucose	Yes	No	FG ____ mg · dL^{-1}	Medication	Yes	No
Obesity	Yes	No	BMI ____ kg · m^{-2} Waist ____ cm			
Physical Inactivity	Yes	No	Vig. PA 20 min/ 3 days Yes No	Mod. PA 30 min/ 5 days Yes No		
High HDL	Yes	No				

Signs or symptoms of cardiovascular/pulmonary disease (check all that apply):

____ chest discomfort   ____ paroxysmal noc. dyspnea   ____ ankle edema

____ shortness of breath   ____ known heart murmur   ____ syncope   ____ none

____ intermittent claudication ____ palpitations/tachycardia   ____ unusual fatigue

---

MEDICAL HISTORY

Cardiac: Yes   No   If yes, explain _____

Pulmonary: Yes   No   If yes, explain _____

Metabolic: Yes   No   If yes, explain _____

List Medications: _____
_____
_____
_____

Risk Stratification (circle one):	**Low Risk**	**Moderate Risk**	**High Risk**

_____   _____

Testing Staff Name   Date

See *Table 2.1* for Risk Factor Thresholds
See *Table 2.2* for Symptoms of Cardiovascular, Pulmonary, or Metabolic Diseases
See *Table 2.3* for Risk Stratification Criteria

BODY COMPOSITION DATA FORM

....

Client Name	Date	Technician(s)	File #

Weight History Review

Weight at age 18 _____ lbs

   Cyclic Wt Loss? Y/N

Recent Wt Loss? Y/N if yes (lbs, time) _____

Previous Body Comp. Data (% fat, wt, date) _____

Visual Impression Record

% fat appearance: (circle one)

   <10   10–15   15–20   20–25   25–30   >30

Overall appearance:

   Lean / Muscular / Average / Fat

Body Comp Considerations:

   Exercise (last 3 hrs): Y/N   Eating (last 3 hrs): Y/N   Void (last 1 hr): Y/N

Height/Weight   Weight (nearest 0.25 lb) ____ lb   /   2.2046 = ____ kg

                    Height (nearest 0.25 in) ____ in   ×   0.0254 = ____ m

                    Body Mass Index (kg · m^{-2}) ____ kg / (____ m × ____ m) = ____

Circumferences (cm)

	1	2	3	Mean	
Waist	____	____	____	____	Waist Hip Ratio: _____
Hip	____	____	____	____	

Skinfolds (mm)

Sex	Site	1	2	3	Mean	
W	Triceps	____	____	____	____	***Body Density: 1.__ __ __**
W	Suprailiac	____	____	____	____	
W	Thigh	____	____	____	____	***%Fat (3 site):** _____
	alternate	____	____	____	____	
M	Chest	____	____	____	____	Staff Comments:_____
M	Abdomen	____	____	____	____	_____
M	Thigh	____	____	____	____	_____

*See below: *3-Site Formula* and *Conversion of Body Density (Db) to Percent Body Fat*

*3-Site *Skinfold Formulas by gender:*

Men: *Body Density = 1.112 − 0.00043499 (SSF__) + 0.00000055 (SSF__)^2 − 0.00028826 (Age__)*

Women: *Body Density = 1.097 − 0.00046971 (SSF__) + 0.00000056 (SSF__)^2 − 0.00012828*
                   (Age__)

*Body Density (Db) to *Percent Body Fat Conversion by age/gender:*

Men ages 20–80yrs.: *(4.95/Db) − 4.50*

Women ages 20–80yrs.: *(5.01/Db) − 4.57*

Staff Comments: _____

_____

_____

MUSCULAR FITNESS DATA FORM

_____   _____   _____   _____

Client Name   Date   Technician(s)   File #

Age: _____   Gender: _____   Weight: _____ lb _____ kg Height: _____ in _____ cm

Strength Assessment

Right Hand Grip Strength

Trial 1 (kg)   Trial 2 (kg)   Trial 3 (kg)   **Best Score (kg)**
_____   _____   _____   _____

Left Hand Grip Strength

Trial 1 (kg)   Trial 2 (kg)   Trial 3 (kg)   **Best Score (kg)**
_____   _____   _____   _____

Combined Score: _____   Classification: _____

1-RM Bench Press Strength

Trial 1 (kg)   Trial 2 (kg)   Trial 3 (kg)   **Best Score (kg)**   **Ratio**
_____   _____   _____   _____   _____

Classification: _____

1-RM Leg Press Strength

Trial 1 (kg)   Trial 2 (kg)   Trial 3 (kg)   **Best Score (kg)**   **Ratio**
_____   _____   _____   _____   _____

Classification: _____

Endurance Assessment

YMCA Submaximal Bench Press

Total Number of Lifts _____
Classification: _____

Push-Up Test

Total Number of Push-ups _____
Classification: _____

Curl-Up Test

Total Number of Curl-ups _____
Classification: _____

FLEXIBILITY DATA FORM

....

_____   _____   _____   _____
Client Name   Date   Technician(s)   File #

Age: _____   Gender: _____   Weight: _____ lb _____ kg   Height: _____ in _____ cm

Sit and Reach Test

Trial 1 (in)   Trial 2 (in)   Trial 3 (in)   **Best Score (in)**
_____   _____   _____   _____

'Zero'Point: _____ Inches   Classification: _____

Sit and Reach Test

Trial 1 (cm)   Trial 2 (cm)   Trial 3 (cm)   **Best Score (cm)**
_____   _____   _____   _____

'Zero'Point: _____ cm   Classification: _____

Lumbar Extension Test

Trial 1 (in)   Trial 2 (in)   Trial 3 (in)   **Best Score (in)**
_____   _____   _____   _____

Classification: _____

Lumbar Flexion Test

Trial 1 (in)   Trial 2 (in)   Trial 3 (in)   **Best Score (in)**
_____   _____   _____   _____

Classification: _____

Range of Motion Assessments.

Flexibility Test	Measured Range of Motion
Shoulder Flexion	
Shoulder Extension	
Shoulder Internal Rotation	
Shoulder External Rotation	
Hip Flexion (testing leg fully extended)	
Hip Flexion (testing knee flexed 90° and hip flexed 90°)	
Hip Extension (testing leg fully extended)	
Hip Abduction	
Hip Adduction	

SUBMAXIMAL CYCLE TEST DATA FORM

Name: _____ Age: _____ Sex: _____ Date: _____

Time of test: _____ ID #: _____

Rest HR: _____ Rest BP: _____
         supine / sitting*   supine / sitting*

Weight: _____ lb _____ kg Height: _____ in _____ cm

RISK STRATIFICATION: _____

Hours since last meal? _____ List food and/or beverages: _____

MEDICATIONS: Dose   Time last taken

_____

_____

_____

_____

ACTIVITY/EXERCISE HISTORY: _____

PAST ET: Date: _____ HR$_{max}$: _____ BP$_{max}$: _____/_____ $\dot{V}O_{2max}$: _____ Test Time: _____ Protocol: _____

Minute	Resistance (kg)	kg · m · min^{-1}	Pulse Palpation (15 s)	HR Monitor (bpm)	BP (mm Hg)	RPE
1						
2						
3						
4						
5						
6						
7						
8						
9						
10						
11						
12						
Recovery 1						
Recovery 2						
Recovery 3						

Estimated $\dot{V}O_{2max}$: _____

Fitness Classification: _____

EXERCISE TEST DATA FORM

Name: _____ Age: _____ Sex: _____ Date: _____

Time of test: _____ ID #: _____

Rest HR: _____   Rest BP: _____
            supine / sitting*   supine / sitting*

Weight: _____ lb _____ kg   Height: _____ in _____ cm

RISK STRATIFICATION: _____

Hours since last meal? _____ List food and/or beverages: _____

MEDICATIONS: Dose   Time last taken
_____
_____
_____

ACTIVITY/EXERCISE HISTORY: _____

PAST ET: Date: _____ HR_{max}: _____ BP_{max}: _____/_____ $\dot{V}O_{2max}$: _____ Test Time: _____ Protocol: _____

Protocol: _____

Time (min)	Work setting	HR (bpm)	BP (mm HG)	RPE	Comments
0–1	/		/		
1–2	/		/		
2–3	/		/		
3–4	/		/		
4–5	/		/		
5–6	/		/		
6–7	/		/		
7–8	/		/		
8–9	/		/		
9–10	/		/		
10–11	/		/		
11–12	/		/		
12–13	/		/		
13–14	/		/		
14–15	/		/		

Immediate Post-Test Symptoms:	Chest Discomfort	SOB	Lightheadedness	Other
RECOVERY			**ACTIVE or SUPINE**	
0–1		/		
1–2		/		
2–3		/		
3–4		/		
4–5		/		

REASON for STOPPING TEST: _____

TECH 1: _____ TECH 2: _____ SUPERVISOR: _____
_____

Note: work setting is speed and grade for the treadmill or resistance and rpms for the cycle.
*Use standing for a treadmill test.

Index

Page numbers followed by *b*, *f*, or *t* indicate boxed, figures, or table material.